Lawful Exit

Lawful Exit

The limits of freedom
for help in dying

Derek Humphry

The Norris Lane
Press

Published by
The Norris Lane Press
Junction City, OR 97448-9559
USA
Telephone and FAX: 503/998-1873

Distributed by
BookWorld Services, Inc.
1933 Whitfield Loop
Sarasota, FL 34243
Phone: 800/444-2524 anytime
Fax: 813/753-9396

ISBN 0-9637280-0-8

Library of Congress Catalog Card Number 93-92721

Other books by Derek Humphry

General
Because They're Black
Police Power and Black People
Passports and Politics
False Messiah
The Cricket Conspiracy
Euthanasia
Jean's Way
Let Me Die Before I Wake: How dying people end their suffering
The Right to Die: Understanding euthanasia
Final Exit: Self-deliverance and assisted suicide for the dying
Dying with Dignity
Work in Progress:
Seesaw: An autobiography

Research for this book
by Abby Gleicher

The author's thanks for criticisms and suggestions to: Faye J. Girsh, Ed.D.; Robert L Risley, J.D; The Reverend John R. Brooke; Midge Levy; Betty and Des Pengelly; Lee D Kersten, J.D; Professor Charles Baron; Karen Cooper; Nancy Dorfman; Don L. Parker; Cheryl K Smith, J.D; Samuel I Sigal, J.D; Griffith D. Thomas, M.D. J.D; Trish Hooper; John Foss; Luis A. Gallop; David B Clarke, J.D., and Gerald A. Larue.

For my loyal friend Jean Holmes Gillett

A desire to terminate one's own life is probably the ultimate exercise of one's right to privacy.

-- Judges in the case of *Bouvia v. Supreme Court*

Freedom is the right to choose: the right to create for yourself the alternatives of choice. Without the possibility of choice and the exercise of choice a man is not a man but a member, an instrument, a thing.

-- Archibald MacLeish, poet.

I shall not abandon old age, if old age preserves me intact as regards the better part of myself; but if old age begins to shatter my mind, and to pull its various faculties to pieces, if it leaves me, not life, but only the breath of life, I shall rush out of a house that is crumbling and tottering. I shall not avoid illness by seeking death, as long as the illness is curable and does not impede my soul. I shall not lay violent hands upon myself just because I am in pain; for death under such circumstances is defeat. But if I find out that the pain must always be endured, I shall depart, not because of the pain, but because it will be a hindrance to me as regards all my reasons for living.

--Seneca *c* 3 BC - AD 65

The author

Derek Humphry was a journalist and author in Britain for 30 years. He worked for the *Daily Mail* and *Sunday Times*, specializing in race relations, civil liberties and the civil war in Northern Ireland. His books of that period include *Because They're Black,* which won the 1972 Martin Luther King Memorial Prize.

In 1978 he moved to America to work for the *Los Angeles Times*. At the same time his account of helping his terminally ill wife to die, *Jean's Way*, was published in both countries and launched him on a campaign for the right of the terminally ill to have lawful access to euthanasia. In 1980 he founded the Hemlock Society and as executive director until 1992 he helped it grow to 57,000 members and 91 chapters. He was president of the World Federation of Right to Die Societies from 1988-1990 and still serves on its board as newsletter editor. He is also vice-president of Americans for Death With Dignity.

Lawful Exit is his sixth book on euthanasia over 15 years. It is the sequel to his most famous book, *Final Exit,* which remained 18 weeks on the *New York Times* best seller list in 1991 and was translated into eleven languages.

Derek and his wife Gretchen live in the hills of western Oregon, gardening and sailing for relaxation. He can be contacted through P O Box 10603, Eugene, OR 97440-2603.

CONTENTS

Glossary of Terms

Euthanasia. Help with a good death. (Legally vague but useful as a broad, descriptive term.)

Passive euthanasia. The deliberate disconnection of life support equipment, or cessation of any medical procedure, permitting the death of a patient.

Physician aid-in-dying. Action by a medical doctor to end the life of a patient by either of the next two definitions.

Active voluntary euthanasia. The action of one person directly helping another to die on request. (For instance, a physician agreeing to give a terminal patient a lethal injection.)

Assisted suicide. Providing the means by which a person can take his or her own life. (For example, a physician writing a prescription or supplying a lethal drug knowing that this is meant for the person to cause their own death)

Kill. To deprive a person or creature of life.

Murder/Homicide. Unlawfully slaying a person who wished to live.

Suicide. Ending one's life.

Self-deliverance. A person irreversibly ill who makes a rational decision to end his or her own life. This term is preferred by those who consider that equating this action with "suicide" to be inaccurate and unfair.

Rational Suicide. Ending one's own life for considered reasons as opposed to emotional or psychological ones.

Silent suicide. Starving oneself to death. Usually carried out in extreme old age.

Mercy killing Ending another person's life without his or her request in the belief that it is a compassionate act. (This term is usually applied to a violent action such as shooting.)

Heroic measures. Medical procedures which are pointless because the person is certain to die.

Double effect. Giving drugs to a patient to relieve pain while at the same time recognizing these may hasten death.

Negotiated death. An agreement between family and physicians (including hospital management and attorneys for both sides) that life support systems to an incompetent person will be disconnected at a certain point in the best interests of the patient. All parties agree not to bring lawsuits.

Snow (slang). To administer heavy doses of narcotics to sedate a person dying painfully.

C P R (Cardiopulmonary resuscitation). Non-surgical massage of a heart which has stopped to try to get the organ working again. Procedure will almost always be started unless there is a D N R order.

D N R (Do not resuscitate). An order on the patient's medical chart advising health professionals that extraordinary measures should not be used to attempt to save the person's life.

Slow code (or Code Blue). The deliberate slow response to a medical alert of heart or breathing stoppage designed to make resuscitation impossible.

Advance directives. Legally accurate name for the next two documents.

Living Will. Popular name for an advance directive by which a person requests a physician not to connect, or to disconnect, life-support equipment if this procedure is merely delaying an inevitable death.

Durable Power of Attorney for Health Care. An advance directive by which a person nominates another person to make health care decisions if and when he/she is incompetent, thus allowing by proxy decision a treating physician to obtain informed consent to a medical procedure or refusal of treatment.

Health Care Proxy. Same as above. This name is used in Massachusetts and New York.

Terminal illness. The condition of a sick person for which there is no apparent cure.

Irreversibly ill. Another way of saying terminally ill.

Hopelessly ill. Patient with a disease which has no known cure but is not immediately life-threatening.

Ethics. A system of moral standards or values.

Medical Ethicist. Person with philosophical and/or legal training who offers opinions on moral matters which confront physicians and psychiatrists.

Hospice A formal program of palliative care for persons in the last six months of life, providing pain management, symptom control, and family support.

Palliative care. Medical term for hospice. Measures which do not attempt to treat the illness but to relieve the pain and other discomfort accompanying it.

Right to die. Popular general term reflecting a basic belief that end of life decisions should be a person's choice.

Right to choose to die. A more accurate term for the above.

Right to life. Popular general term for belief that death should only come about by the will of a deity, or the belief that life is the prevailing value, regardless of conditions or desires to end it for whatever reason.

Slippery slope. Theory that the sanctioning of an act that, in itself, may not be morally repugnant or illegal but could lead to other acts which are.

Persistent Vegetative State. Brain-damaged person in a permanent coma from which they are not likely to recover. Has no cognitive functions.

Brain damage. Injury to the brain causing impairment. Life support systems optional.

Coma. Prolonged unconsciousness, from which a person may recover.

Brain death. Complete cessation of cognitive function. Life support systems useless.

Cortex. The outer layer of gray matter over most of the brain.

I C U. Intensive care unit.

Miracle cure. A sudden healing occasioned by a deity or a medical discovery. Rare.

Trauma. An accident or incident that affects body or mind.

Competent/competency. The ability of a person to communicate with a physician and understand the implications and consequences of medical procedures.

Informed consent. A patient giving permission to a physician to carry out a medical procedure after he/she is made fully aware of the benefits, risks and any alternatives.

Note: I accept that some of my definitions have possible alternatives. But until we try to speak a common language about "death and dying" there will be misunderstandings and the debate will be flawed.

Introduction

Individual freedom requires that all persons be allowed to control their own destiny, especially at life's end. Existing law does not permit this basic right. Therefore, the law must be reformed to permit a terminally ill patient the right to request and receive the assistance of a physician in dying. The reformed law must protect those who willingly provide assistance, and it must protect society against abuse.

For those who believe in the right to choose to die and wish a physician to help them, the requirements are quite simple:

A thoughtfully framed law which enables the patient to ask for death, and a willing physician to be able to provide the means, without fear of prosecution, persecution, or stigma.

This is the ultimate civil liberty, the freedom to select one's own manner of dying without interference from others, but with help if we choose. If we cannot die by our choice, then we are not free people. Those who want this choice do not seek to impose our views on others who have different ethical perspectives. Freedom of choice means just that: to each his own. They do not wish to trap unwilling physicians into helping people to die if it offends their professional or moral codes. But for those people and physicians who know that sometimes it is morally right to assist the death of a hopelessly ill person at their rational request, action is required to reform existing laws that prohibit this.

Many people ask me, "Why is it proving so difficult for a civilized society to allow dying persons the option of release from unbearable suffering? After all, we do it for our pets and our farm animals."

I never advance the 'pets have euthanasia' argument because the animal kingdom is not surrounded with thousands of years of taboos and laws connected with death and dying. Whether my dog is healthy or sick, I can lawfully kill it if I wish so long as I do it humanely. But I cannot kill another human being unless ordered into war by my government, can prove self-defense, or am the appointed executioner of a judicially condemned prisoner. Animals do not have choice in dying. Nevertheless, the 'pets have euthanasia' argument is significant if you are a person who considers that a society's moral values can be judged by how that society cares for its dumb animals which have no established rights.

It is proving a tough fight to change the laws on the right to die because certain religious orders with considerable financial clout do not ethically approve of a human being having individual control over what happens to their bodies, and because the leaders of the medical profession traditionally resist reform of the customs and practices of their profession.

The religious right will not be changed. However word-perfect and abuse-free the *Death With Dignity Act* is made, they will not be convinced. This is not the intent. Let the members of the religious right die in their chosen fashion. But to avoid their stultifying attitudes the medical profession must be offered a law it feels comfortable with.

The evidence is now overwhelming that at least half of the medical profession in America-- and probably in other countries, as well-- supports a change in the law to allow patients to request help in ending their lives under special conditions. When thinking about physicians dealing with death, we have to remind ourselves that a great many have nothing at all to do with the subject. They work in specialties where patients are not terminally ill. Yet their views on euthanasia are just as influential in the corridors of medical power as those of a physician with a geriatric or oncology practice who deals with death every day.

If one listens at conferences of physicians and nurses, particularly those concerned with intensive care, it is obvious that euthanasia in many forms is currently being practiced covertly in American hospitals. "It happens every day in ICUs," some health workers say. Nurses tell me that they have no qualms about deliberately overdosing some patients who are close to death, with or without their permission, because the suffering is so great and death does not come soon enough as a release. Two nurses in the presence of eight other physicians and nurses who nodded agreement stated, "There's not an ICU in the country which is not practicing euthanasia but we don't call it that. We prefer not to call it anything. We know in our hearts that the person really died of the underlying sickness, not the bolus of morphine which we just injected."

Because they are affected by seeing in the course of their work the very worst aspects of dying, a great many physicians and nurses have private agreements between themselves that they will hasten each others' deaths should they be unfortunate enough to resemble the condition of some of their patients. "Nurses have a clear sense of when enough is enough for a patient," an experienced nursing instructor told me. A famous American physician has said publicly that he hopes that he will know soon enough if he is getting

21

Alzheimer's disease so that he can kill himself before he becomes what he termed "a human vegetable."

What I have reported here begs the question that if beneficent euthanasia is being so widely practiced, why then do we need to reform the law? First, it is written into most laws that assisting death in any circumstance is a crime. And then, for every suffering patient who gets an assisted death from a courageous physician or nurse, another may suffer because their particular caregivers are either afraid of breaking the law or are opposed (as they are entitled to be) on religious or ethical grounds to hastening death. There have been occasional instances where a "born-again" nurse reports to her or his superiors that colleagues have been overdosing dying patients. Fear that this might happen deters some physicians and nurses from being angels of mercy. "If our superiors knew what we were doing, that would be the end for us," said a physician.

Without a law in place, there are no criteria or guidelines (in hospital jargon, "protocols") for these secretive actions. Abuse is always possible. It is also extremely unfair to ask physicians and nurses to take solitary responsibility for these onerous decisions by not altering the law to accommodate and control the practice. Hypocritically ignoring or defying existing laws, or being too lazy to modify them, demeans the whole rule of law under which our civilization exists.

The right to die movement has made huge strides in the past twenty years. But resistance from those who oppose choice is stiffening. Then there is Dr. Kevorkian. Few would deny that the 16 sick people who went to him between 1990 and early 1993 to be helped to die were deserving of his assistance as their ultimate choice. But his defiance of the law has caused a backlash in many parts of America. His own state has now made it a crime to assist a suicide under any circumstances. Up until then, attempts to prosecute Dr. Kevorkian failed through lack of a clear legal prohibition. This means that other physicians in Michigan who might have been willing to help certain patients die are now handicapped. So great is the fear that Dr. Kevorkian will move his activities to their territory that legislation was introduced in early 1993 in seven other states making it criminal to assist a suicide under any circumstance, with stiff punishments. Some of these states previously had merely classified the action as a "misdemeanor" with extremely light penalties. Whether any of the seven states will succeed in actually passing the new laws remains to be seen, of course, but if Michigan is any bellwether, some will. The states where this is happening are Connecticut, Georgia, Indiana, North Carolina, Ohio, South Carolina, and Tennessee.

Dr. Kevorkian has stated publicly that he will continue to assist suicides of dying people despite Michigan's ban, and risk prosecution. Considering that more than 6,000 people die every day in the USA, the 16 people whom Dr. Kevorkian has helped over nearly three years could be seen as largely symbolic (which is not to detract from their needs). Undoubtedly his well-publicized actions have aroused enormous public debate, which is healthy, but his disregard for law and law reform, his extremely slender medical credentials, and the cursory acquaintance he has with his clients before they die, have earned him severe criticism as well.

If legislation permitting justifiable voluntary euthanasia is not passed soon, people and groups will increasingly take the law into their own hands. Then Dr. Kevorkian's scale of operations will be dwarfed. This frustration is already evidenced by the start-up in Washington State of a service providing on-call, home-visiting assisted suicide which does not use the services of physicians, but relies instead on experienced lay people. This is merely a half-way step because, if euthanasia is to be practiced with dignity and certainty, a physician has to be involved.

The purpose of this book is to help frame a sensible law which we who revere personal freedom can understand and support. We need to look back at the history of *The Death With Dignity Act*, to review its development since 1985, and rewrite it giving equal weight to the rights of both patients and physicians. At the same time, we must not erect so many hurdles that it is next to impossible for the dying patient to surmount them.

Chapter 1

Time to change

Forty-six percent of the electors in two American states, Washington and California, voted affirmatively when asked if they wanted to change the law to permit physicians to agree to the requests of terminally ill people to be helped to die, a total of 5,263,828 people. This was a higher percentage vote than put President Clinton into office. If laws were changed on a county basis, the entire Bay area of San Francisco would now have lawful euthanasia. However, for voters' initiatives to pass, they must win 51 percent of the total vote statewide. So we are left with this question: would the law have passed if it had been better written, dispelling the natural doubts and fears people have when deciding on a significant social change? Across the nation, indeed, across the world, public opinion polls asking this question in many different ways reach a consensus of approximately 70 percent of people backing physician-aided dying in principle but, of course, not in law.

The difference between winning and losing in the two West coast states was the failure to convince the medical profession that *The Death With Dignity Act* had sufficient protections against abuse, both by physicians and families. A section of the public which had previously expressed positive views about the new law sensed that physicians were uneasy about it and withheld their support at the polls.

The fact that the combined might of the Roman

25

Catholic, fundamentalist and evangelical churches spent millions fighting the proposed law would not have made the difference had the proponents been able confidently to respond: "Ah! But physicians agree with us." The legislation specifically excluded private hospitals from having to obey the proposed law, but Catholic hospitals, for whom this exemption was inserted, still poured thousands of dollars into the "No" campaign. For them, as for the rest of the churches which opposed, it was a matter of morality: theirs. The religious right holds that people who think and act differently than they should not be allowed to-- a curious philosophy in a nation which was historically founded upon the freedom of religion, and freedom from other people's religions.

Therefore to pass into law the right of freedom of choice in dying requires a partnership between the supporting public and the supporting medical profession. Turning to Dr. Kevorkian or buying *Final Exit* is stopgap, really not adequate unless a person is dying in an unbearable fashion at this moment. Civilized people in the future need a clearly-defined situation where there is trust and respect between a dying patient and the physician so that the appropriate medical action is taken in particular circumstances, with neither party at risk of legal or financial punishment.

Those who want this freedom of choice to die in a manner and by a means which is right for them are obliged to reform the law because the universal sanction against assistance in death is firmly enshrined in the majority of current laws. The taboo has been stripped away in the past 15 years by the proliferation of right-to-die groups, and public shock over certain "mercy killing" cases, two "how-to" suicide books, and so-called "Dr. Death" in Michigan, but the criminal prohibition in the law remains unaltered. While Dr. Kevorkian has proved his point that desperately ill dying people want the services of a physician in suicide, he ridiculed the two West coast law reform campaigns and also succeeded in provoking his own state to renew its ban on assisted suicide. Thus he has made it harder for some patients to get their doctors to discreetly assist them to die.

The long-standing criminal sanction against assistance in suicide stems from the 2,000 year-old Judeo-Christian belief in the sanctity of life. One of the ten commandments says, "Thou shalt not kill." And that rule has been interpreted to include killing oneself, self-murder. Christianity has such a long history of bloody battles fought in its name, of burning heretics at the stake, and of condoning capital punishment that I wonder about the true meaning of this commandment.

Thankfully, most people nowadays do not directly connect law with religion. The criminality of all forms of assisted suicide is a unfortunate holdover from the days when religious morality influenced law making. Suicide used to be a crime in many places, punishable by giving the estate of the dead person to the monarch or feudal lord and depriving the heirs. When I was a cub reporter on a local newspaper in England in the 1950s there was a sad procession through the courts which I was reporting of miserable people charged with criminal attempted suicide. I never saw one sent to prison, only ordered to have psychological care. This charade ceased in 1961 when Britain led the way in decriminalizing suicide and attempted suicide but here, too, assisted suicide was written into the code as a crime punishable by up to 14 years' imprisonment. Most American states do not make suicide or attempted suicide a crime (in the few states which do, the law

27

lies in abeyance) but continue to make assisted suicide a crime. Those which do not have a specific statute could charge it as manslaughter or second-degree murder. The universal prohibition on assisted suicide was originally installed to protect unstable people from getting help in self-destruction, and also to uphold the states' duty to protect life. When these laws were passed, no consideration was given to the right-to-die of terminally ill persons-- this has only been a big issue since the mid-1970s.

Thus what the pro-euthanasia movement has embarked upon is a campaign of modernization of the obsolescent laws relating to the sanctity of life. Life is sacred. But we deny its sacral quality when we let life degenerate to a point where it becomes unbearable and meaningless for the individual and we do nothing to help. In the end, it comes down to the issue of quality of life compared to quantity of life. Which does a person want? Both individual choices must be respected. (Assisted suicide for evil or reckless reasons should remain a crime)

Voluntariness has to be the quintessence of euthanasia legislation. Without it we are as bad as the Nazis who forced nearly 100,000 of their own people who were handicapped, physically or mentally, into the gas chambers. The Nazi propaganda apparatus cleverly called it "euthanasia" as a coverup tactic for wholesale murder. Voluntariness must be built like a rock into all legislation. Voluntary for the patient to request lethal drugs and voluntary for the physician to agree or refuse to help. What distinguishes what I am advocating in contrast to what the Nazis did is the considered personal choice of an adult who is nearing certain death. In Hitler's genocidal world it was murder as defined in my glossary.

28

For whom is euthanasia available?

Under the uniform model *Death With Dignity Act* at the back of this book, the only person who can be helped by a willing physician to die is an adult who is terminally ill, appears likely to die within the next six months, and has the mental capacity to understand both the consequences of asking for assisted death and any alternatives.

No mention is made in the law of the degree of suffering or quality of life. These are subjective matters, but they must be thoroughly dealt with in the guidelines which accompany the law. People have different thresholds of pain and varying criteria for quality of life decisions. If physicians were asked to make legal judgment calls on the extent of a patient's suffering, it could be embarrassing to both. We must assume that patients are not likely to ask for hastened death unless they are in pain and/or distress. Remember, to qualify they must be suffering from a physical illness which in an advanced terminal state.

The benefits of *The Death With Dignity Act* are not confined to the actual help in dying. Persons in early stages of terminal illness will gain comfort from the knowledge that there is euthanasia to fall back on should their suffering eventually become intolerable. This may help them bear the pain and indignities for the duration of their illness. Additionally, acceptance that death is coming-- whether in the outcome it turns out to be either natural or induced-- enables a terminally ill person to tidy up business and domestic affairs, say the important goodbyes, and close out any unfinished business and unresolved conflicts. In the Netherlands, about 25,000 people a year with terminal illnesses initially ask their physicians about

29

the possibility of euthanasia, but eventually only about 3,000 actually receive it. The others either did not need it, changed their minds, died before it became available, or were refused by physicians (*Remmelink Report*).

I am not alone in this belief: that to have the knowledge that one can bring to an end his own life, painlessly, through the appropriate use of euthanasia is, in fact, life affirming. If people are confident that there is an "escape hatch" then they may feel able to accept some of the pain and distress, even risk untried therapies, with a chance of a longer life.

The ground-breaking legislation which this book proposes, when passed will demand more of physicians than they have been giving patients over the past 40 years. Such a sensitive and complex law involving the irredeemable act of assisting death, will require that the medical profession trains young physicians better in matters of ethics and law. It will force physicians to relate more intimately with their patients by spending more time with them and understanding patient problems. It will slow the trend in modern medicine for physicians to be highly specialized body technicians and steer them towards being healing artists with a human touch. Technology and medical science will be relegated to its proper place as a valuable assistant to health care but no longer the dominating factor. We shall see more physicians at the deathbed, a practice which they have largely abandoned in contemporary times. Physicians will have to be much more knowledgeable and careful, which can only resound to the profession's benefit.

Who cannot get help to die?

30

Physician aid-in-dying is not available under *The Death With Dignity Act* to people in the early stages of terminal illness. Modern medicine, and particularly pain control, are so sophisticated these days that quite often life can be usefully extended and still have reasonable quality. Some diseases move faster than expected; many others move slower after treatment, especially if detected early on. This law is not designed to allow anybody to throw away part of their lives which have at least some value. Nor is it fair to ask physicians to help end lives unless the prognosis is desperate and painful.

It is not available to people who are dying but are unconscious, or lack the capacity to understand anything a physician says to them. This is a sad omission which I regret. But the many complexities of writing a law at present that would include helping them to die are extremely controversial. For the time being we must discriminate against the incompetent person in order to bring quicker help to the competent terminally ill. When *The Death With Dignity Act* is running smoothly, and we have learned how to practice euthanasia, then society should address the vexing question of how patients could get help with death even though they are incompetent in their final days. The basic ingredient obviously must be a clear advance directive made while the capacity to think still exists.

Minors are not included. Most deaths of children are by accident; the lingering, painful deaths are chiefly reserved for the over 50's. It has not come to my attention that there is a significant problem with the deaths of those under 18, although I grant that there must be exceptions. Laws governing the care of children are, of course, infinitely different from

31

those of adults and to mingle the two age groups in one law--
even were it necessary-- would cause endless problems.

The depressed and the mentally ill cannot get help to die
under this law. Many intelligent and caring people have made
the case to me over the years that the suffering of mental
illness can be every bit as painful as terminal cancer, and even
from my slender experience in the field of psychology, I
believe them. Quite a few people hold that persons with acute
mental illness which has not responded to treatment deserve the
choice of euthanasia. Quite frankly, that is a minefield across
which I do not choose to walk. The chance of misdiagnosis,
the possibility of successful treatment or cure, or the risk of a
hoax could cause this to blow up in the face of those who
practiced it. Persons who are severely mentally ill are often
suffering pure hell, and if their only relief is suicide then I
respect that choice. I would not stop a severely mentally sick
person who had spent years in treatment from ending it all, but
neither would I help the action, nor encourage anybody else to
do so. Countless numbers of people throughout history have
escaped the torture of mental illness by suicide and-- though we
should always try our best to understand and to treat their pain-
- it will continue until the working of the human brain is fully
understood. Persons suffering from depression for whatever
reasons are similarly excluded from using *The Death With
Dignity Act*-- the essential qualification is a life-threatening
physical illness.

The rate of suicide among the elderly is soaring
worldwide. In 1990 United States statistics, the old comprised
12.5% of the population and committed 20.7% of suicides.
Surveys show that the most likely reason for an older person to

self-destruct is deteriorating health, with loneliness, grief, and psychological problems close behind. Should a person in his 70s or 80s who has serious medical problems which are not responding to treatment be helped to die if he makes considered and persistent requests? A good many senior citizens believe they deserve this option and I have never hidden the fact that I agree with them. But at this point in time neither society nor the medical profession is willing to legislate this right to the seniors so I have not included it in *The Death With Dignity Act*. I predict that it will be available early in the next century as the world population ages and more attention is paid to geriatric problems by the succeeding generation.

The right to life movement claims that "the right to die will become the duty to die." They hold that when euthanasia is institutionalized, the ailing elderly will start to feel obligated to the younger generations to get out of the way to spare expense and trouble. This is a doom-laden argument, taking no account of the love that most families feel for their old folks. True, some families are uncaring for their seniors, but they are the exception. When did exceptions ever create the rule? The "duty to die" argument takes no account of the vociferousness of senior citizens and their acknowledged voting power. Far more seniors involve themselves in community affairs and politics than do younger generations. I cannot believe that being 70 or 80 years old, with a euthanasia law on the statute, automatically means a person is going to allow the family to push them into the grave. The will to live is too potent.

Severely physically disabled people such as paraplegics and quadriplegics also do not qualify for assistance under *The Death With Dignity Act*. Remarkable few "quads" want to end their existences, preferring courageously to find meaning to their lives in a multitude of ways. There are a few exceptions, but laws are passed to benefit society as a whole and not the occasional individual. I have known some severely disabled people who found their handicaps unbearable and preferred death. Either they found ways to kill themselves alone or had good friends-- sometimes even parents-- who helped. These cases deserve our understanding and mercy but do not justify a law.

Even tougher are decisions about people who are hopelessly ill and for whose complaint there is no effective treatment. They face often many years of physical and mental agony. Severe arthritis is perhaps the most common example. The letters describing their ordeals are the most harrowing I receive. Alzheimer's Disease and Multiple Sclerosis are among the degenerative diseases from which three out of every five people will die in modern civilization. Who is to say that a person with an unchallengeable diagnosis of Alzheimers or MS does not have the right to decide to refuse to spend years dying? Should not such people be able to avoid the distress, indignities and the emotional and financial strains it puts on their families? We all hope for a cure to be found for these diseases but I cannot find it in my heart to condemn a person who, at a fairly advanced stage of their disease, decides not to wait any longer for a "miracle cure" as yet unavailable.

The bottom line is whether patients who are irreversibly ill but not imminently dying should be entitled to physician-assisted death. Perhaps so, but the medical profession is not ready for that quantum leap which means there is no point in including such a provision within *The Death With Dignity Act*. This type of patient should be left free to end their own life if that is their choice. In the next century society and the medical profession will be more tolerant of this category of chosen death.

Referring to the future, of course, is where we must tackle the matter of the so-called "slippery slope." All social progress comes in stages. Divorce used to be only for the wealthy because of the many restrictions placed upon the procedure; nowadays marriages of the rich and poor alike are ended by mutual consent. Abortion used to be only for critical medical reasons; now it is upon a woman's demand, with some criteria. All homosexual behavior used to be punishable but today, within reason, it is acceptable. Suicide and attempted suicide, as I have said, used to be crimes but today they are not, while assistance in suicide remains a crime. Anybody who doubts that in the next century there will be much more sympathy for choices in dying than exists today is turning a blind eye to the lessons of history.

The "slippery slope" would be an evil possibility if a government ruthlessly modified a successful *Death With Dignity Act*, passed by popular vote, into a mechanism for killing the poor, the disabled, the elderly, or anybody else it considered "undesirable." But that is not how democracies work. People would not let it happen. When the Act is passed, the searchlight of critical opinion upon it will be so great that any abuses or unapproved modifications will be pounced upon. The Netherlands example proves this point. A person who fears the "slippery slope" has no confidence in our democratic system with its checks and balances. For once, opponents in the right to life movement will play an essential and welcome part in monitoring the implementation and the future of *The*

Death With Dignity Act.

With euthanasia, as with any social progress, lines are drawn. For people who use pornography it is available, but society does not permit X-rated bookstores in residential districts where they would be more easily available to the curiosity of our children. Today a viewer can see the sexual act on a television or cinema screen, but not the sexual organs. A myriad of laws relating to health, food, and human behavior all govern what we may or may not do. And so with euthanasia laws. They will define to what degree society thinks the terminally ill deserve help to die. It remains every citizen's duty to see that the laws are obeyed and never altered without popular consent.

Who performs euthanasia?

I helped my first wife, Jean, to die in 1975 when she was suffering from advanced bone cancer. Jean took her own life and I provided the drugs, sat beside her, and gave her moral support. But we had the backing, so to speak, of a physician. Without that we would have been in a desperate situation. At her suggestion I did not ask the treating physicians for help but went to a man with whom I had worked in journalism who was a physician. Once he was satisfied that he knew the details of the case he provided me with the lethal substances.

It is extremely difficult for a terminally ill person to end his or her life without the support, either directly or sometime later, of a physician. Crucially, they are the only persons with lawful access to lethal drugs. Secondly, physicians are-- or should be-- the patients' advisors on the state of the illness and what the future holds for them. As my model law outlines, nothing is completely certain in medicine, but a physician's specialized knowledge offers a good idea of the future course of the disease, thus giving the patient more information to draw on in making decisions.

Helping some patients to die is part of good medical practice. There must be an express request from the patient and the medical circumstances must be so serious as to justify a physician helping. The argument that "doctors are healers, not killers" is a shallow one because dying is part of the cycle of birth, life, and death, and it is an integral part of a physician's work to alleviate suffering during both the birth and the dying processes. At a certain point, in some terminal cases, physicians run out of procedures which will help. At this point helping the patient to die is the only alternative-- if that is what the patient wants. Of course, if the physician is morally opposed to assisting death then he or she should hand the case to a colleague who is not.

Now, us consider this argument: that giving patients the right to have a physician's help in ending their lives upon request will destroy the trust and confidence which must exist between physician and patient. Opponents claim that patients would tremble in fear every time their physicians gave them an injection, even a flu shot! In the mid-1980s there was a story going around that elderly patients in the Netherlands were afraid to drink their orange juice in case it was laced with poison. This argument assumes that many physicians are instinctively murderers. In fact where a few medical men have been imprisoned for murder it has almost always involved problems in their own family. No physician in the USA has ever been convicted of murdering a patient; in Britain there have been several cases, but these were controversial "mercy killings" with little or no punishment involved. As one physician put it: "If you feel you are shortening a person's life, killing a person, then giving a lethal injection is a negative thought. But if you feel the patient is dying and you are assisting the patient in the death they want to go to, then it can be very positive and compassionate."

The opposite of the "loss of trust" claim may be true. Patients who know that their physician is well informed about the law, understands the complexities of the dying process, and may be willing to go "all the way" with their wishes in a crisis, will inspire confidence. Physicians are understandably nervous about the subtleties consequential upon the passage of *The Death With Dignity Act*. There is a fear that many private hospitals will refuse assistance in death, causing the cases to be "dumped" on public hospitals. This would put unfair pressure on the many physicians who agree with euthanasia in principle but do not wish to be categorized as "angels of death" like Dr. Kevorkian. This is a groundless fear because-- if the Dutch experience is any guide-- relatively few people will ask for euthanasia. In any case, the overburdened physician can always refuse.

Listen to Dr. Herbert Cohen, a general practitioner near Rotterdam, who has helped many patients to die over a long period: "Helping patients die is never good medical practice. It's only the best of two bad possibilities. Good medical practice is to cure someone so they can go skiing. People who oppose euthanasia assume the choice is always between dying and living happily ever after. But sometimes it's just a choice between two ways of dying. I do it once every couple of years. It gives me many sleepless nights whenever I do it.

That's the way it should be. If euthanasia ever becomes easy, that's when you should be checked out by somebody."

Much has been written about the definition of "mental competency." With the easy access to psychological services in America this need not be the sole responsibility of the physician. The possibility is sometimes raised that a physician treating a dying patient who has no health insurance might avoid giving him or her chemotherapy or other expensive treatments, instead channeling the patient subtly towards euthanasia. It has been suggested that a physician could give the patient such poor pain control that he or she yearns for death. These are problems which the guidelines must tackle by forbidding such behavior which in properly supervised medicine would be rare. With the 1993 Oregon rationing experiment and President Clinton's commendable emphasis on achieving health care for everybody, the problem of the indigent patient should be eliminated. Every person is entitled to medical care appropriate to their condition. Another physician commented, "If we wait until there is universal access to health care we will hold back forever. Some of us see it (euthanasia) as a silver bullet and the result of poor care, but that's no excuse for denying rational people the help they need to die."

Fears of misdiagnosis are to be found among lay persons but rarely among the medical profession. Is the person really dying? Physicians, of course, like to give the impression that they rarely misdiagnose. Modern medicine is good at testing for problems, even if it is not all that effective at curing them. Physicians are armed now with sophisticated testing equipment, computers, and enjoy easy access to up-to-date medical literature. Thus mistakes are fewer. There is always the second, or third, opinion. A patient with an advanced terminal disease, existing in a body undergoing serious deterioration, and with pain requiring huge amounts of analgesics, hardly needs a physician to tell them death is imminent. What the patient wants to know is, "How long have I got and can you stop the pain?" If people were allowed under *The Death With Dignity Act* to end their lives at the onset of an illness, then misdiagnosis would be a problem. Misdiagnosis right at the end of life is extremely unlikely.

Physicians in big cities like New York and Los Angeles have to treat patients of all races and cultures. Understandably the physician is sometimes baffled by the feelings and value system of a person from another culture with a heritage and religion differing from his own. Might the physician inadvertently steer a confused patient towards a course which he or she really did not want? This is not a problem of euthanasia alone, of course, but it affects all medical treatment which is cross-cultural. In such cases the physician must pause to take skilled advice from neutral observers.

Hospice is the appropriate place, or if being cared for at home, the manner, in which some people die. Unfortunately, America has relatively few stand-alone hospices when compared to Europe. Thus a dying person is most likely to be looked after by visiting physicians and nurses. Pain management, comfort and care, consideration and help with stress on the family, are services which hospice provides admirably. To be admitted to a hospice program the sick person has to be considered likely to die within the next six months, although the average length of care is about one month. If medical care was perfect there would be no need for hospices, which sprang up in the 1970s as a result of serious complaints that physicians were ignorant of pain control techniques and that hospitals were thoughtless and uncaring about the dying process. Although many physicians and hospitals have learned from hospice how to do a better job, there are still too many physicians whose patients would benefit if they were trained in sophisticated pain management.

While I am one of the hospice movement's greatest admirers, it is not the sublime and perfect answer to dying, as some like to claim. Listen to Dr. Timothy Quill, a hospice medical director for eight years: "Those of us who have witnessed difficult deaths of patients on hospice programs are not reassured by the glib assertion that we always know how to make death tolerable, and they fear that physicians will abandon them if their course becomes difficult or overwhelming in the face of comfort care" (*Death and Dignity*, Norton, 1993). Hospice care is not accessible by everybody, either because it is not operating in their district, or because what hospice service is available has to be largely confined to cancer patients. Some in-patient hospices have a religious ethic which may not suit all patients. Every patient must decide whether it is best to perish slowly under excellent care, "snowed' by morphine cocktails, or to select the time, the method, and the style of a self-determined death.

The challenge to society is to pass a law which will enable the small number of patients who are not benefitting from pain management and want euthanasia to be able to get it, while at the same time protecting against abuses. The proposed *Death With Dignity Act* gives no new rights to physicians, but it does give rights to patients. All the Act does for the medical profession is to supply guidelines for action should they choose

41

to help and protection from legal suits.

The thousands of people who worked for, or helped finance, the two failed initiatives in Washington State and California can nevertheless take considerable comfort from the knowledge that many thoughtful physicians and caring hospitals have since worked harder to improve their palliative care services as a response to the voted expression of public disquiet.

Chapter 2

Step by firm step

For real progress towards the legalization of medical assistance in dying, we have of course to look to the Dutch. A progressive yet careful people, they have spent 20 years studying the problems, hammering out the details, and altering-- if not actually the law-- the practice of the law. The Dutch feel that the rule of law exists to serve their purposes and that law must change to suit the times. They have been able to tackle the problems of euthanasia in an open and democratic fashion largely because the Roman Catholic Church in the Netherlands is fairly liberal in its social attitudes. Nor is it the dominant religion. Dutch people are estimated to be one third Protestant, one third Catholic and one third non-religious. There is something deep in the Dutch character which makes them want to solve the problems with which they are confronted; they are a nation which loves commissions of inquiry, academic surveys, erudite conferences, and inter-personal debates far into the night. Then they act. In February of 1993 the Dutch Parliament approved guidelines for euthanasia stopping just short of full legalization. Some argue that this was *de facto* legislation.

How the Dutch reached this intelligent position is worthy of study.

During World War II, the Netherlands was occupied by the Germans for nearly five years. Nazi leaders ordered Dutch physicians to help them carry out their policies of sterilization of Jews, euthanasia of the handicapped, and deportation of Jews and "undesirables" to labor camps. Alone of all the occupied countries, the Dutch medical profession as a group refused to cooperate. The Nazis removed their licenses to practice medicine, but the doctors merely stopped signing birth and death certificates and continued treating patients. Next, the Nazis arrested a sample one hundred physicians and deported them to concentration camps in Germany. Still, the Dutch held firm: no cooperation in any illegal, barbarous policies. Eventually the Nazis gave up. In the end it was the Third Reich's commander, Arthur Seyss-Inquart, known as the "butcher of Holland," who died-- hanged after trial at Nuremburg.

Yet in 1973 the Dutch in combination with the medical profession were the first people in the world to start down the road to lawful voluntary euthanasia for the terminally ill. That year Dr. Geertruida Postma, a general practitioner, was accused of murdering her mother by the injection of morphine. The old lady was in a nursing home, had suffered a cerebral hemorrhage, was partly paralyzed, was being treated for pneumonia, was deaf and spoke only with difficulty. She had failed in a suicide attempt and told her daughter, "I want to leave this life. Please help." At her trial Dr. Postma said her chief regret was not to have done it earlier. Found guilty, her penalty was a one-week suspended sentence and one year of probation. The case woke up the nation. Other physicians declared that they had done the same thing; letters poured into the Minister of Justice; and the Dutch Society for Voluntary Euthanasia was born. It grew into the largest such group in the world.

Over the next twenty years a series of court cases against physicians were brought, more out of a desire to develop an answer than to punish. The most crucial of these cases concerned a physician who had helped a very sick and elderly woman to die, at her request. It went all the way the Dutch Supreme Court, who in 1984 sent it back to the Rotterdam court for a rehearing. This court enunciated what became known as "the Rotterdam criteria" to guide physicians as to when it was appropriate for them to end life.

The same year the Royal Dutch Medical Society announced its approval of justified physician aid-in-dying. Thus the Rotterdam case and blessing of the medical profession brought about a climate for the next nine years in which physicians frequently ended the lives of patients without prosecution. (For a fuller account of the history of Dutch euthanasia, and the Rotterdam criteria, see my book *The Right to Die: Understanding euthanasia*) The flaw in this practice was that the physicians were supposed to fill out extensive reports about the circumstances of the death, and be ready to be interviewed at length by an investigator of the Ministry of Justice if the officials had any doubts. Because they were busy men and woman, some physicians took the short route by signing death certificates giving the underlying cause of death-- such as cancer-- and omitting to say that it was hastened with drugs.

At first, only some dozen cases a year were reported to the Ministry. But as familiarity with procedures grew, so did the reporting: In 1991 there were 590 cases reported; in 1992, over 1,300. As subsequent surveys showed-- somewhere between 2,000 and 3,000 patients were being helped to die annually. The Dutch criminal code said that assisting suicide, or euthanasia, was still a crime. Many people were troubled by the fact that state prosecutors were, in effect, permitting physicians to break the letter of the law. The debate raged on through the late 1980s and early 1990s: should the law be changed or was that step too radical? Would guidelines sanctioned by Parliament suffice? The Royal Dutch Medical Association favored clear legislation in order to protect its members from legal jeopardy. The Dutch Catholic Church, famous for its rejection of many of Rome's dogmas, made no pronouncements for or against, although many individual Catholics protested what they felt was the moral wrongness of what was happening.

By a vote of 91-45 the lower House of Parliament on February 9, 1993, gave immunity to physicians who followed the official guidelines, but declined to strike from the criminal code the penalties for assisted suicide. (Senate and Royal approval followed shortly afterwards. The law takes effect at the beginning of 1994) The reason given for not eliminating the penalties was that if physicians flouted the guidelines then they, like anybody else, would be liable for up to 12 years' imprisonment. Even some Catholic parliamentarians voted for the measure because they felt that this gave the prosecutor a chance to control the practice.

Others, even if they in principle approved of euthanasia, were not happy that the criminal code was not altered. A long-time parliamentary fighter for lawful euthanasia, Jacob Kohnstamm, commented: "This way the legislature is pointing out to doctors how to carefully infringe the law. And the judiciary has to take over the responsibility which the legislature does not want to bear."

My guess, based on watching the way the Dutch operate historically, is that the guidelines, which are given in full here, will be used for about five years, after which point they will have a commission to examine their effectiveness. They will then make any necessary adjustments.

I reprint here the Dutch guidelines in full:

By Order of Parliament
Guidelines for the attending physician in reporting euthanasia to the municipal pathologist in the Netherlands

The following list of points is intended as a guideline in reporting euthanasia or assistance provided to a patient in taking his or her own life to the municipal pathologist. A full written report supplying motives for your action is required.

I. CASE HISTORY

A. What was the nature of the illness and what was the main diagnosis?

B. How long had the patient been suffering from the illness?

C. What was the nature of the medical treatment provided (medication, curative, surgical, etc.)?

D. Please provide the names, addresses and telephone numbers of the attending physicians. What were their diagnoses?

E. Was the patient's mental and/or physical suffering so great that he or she perceived it, or could have perceived it, to be unbearable?

47

F.   Was the patient in a desperate situation with no prospect or relief and was his/her death inevitable?

1.   Was the situation at the end such that the prognosis was increasing lack of dignity for the patient and/or such as to exacerbate suffering which the patient already experienced as unbearable?

2.   Was there no longer any prospect of the patient being able to die with dignity?

3.   When in your opinion would the patient have died if euthanasia had not been performed?

G.   What measures, if any, did you consider or use to prevent the patient experiencing his/her suffering as unbearable (was there indeed any possibility of alleviating the suffering) and did you discuss these with the patient?

II.   REQUEST FOR EUTHANASIA

A.   Did the patient of his/her own free will make a very explicit and deliberate request for euthanasia to be performed:

1.   on the basis of adequate information which you had provided on the course of the illness and the method of terminating life, and

2.   after discussion of the measures referred to at 1G?

B.   If the patient made such a request, when and to whom was it made? Who else was present at the time?

C.   Is there a living will? If so, please pass this on to the municipal pathologist.

D.   At the time of the request was the patient fully aware of the consequences thereof and of his/her physical and mental condition? What evidence of this can you provide?

E.   Did the patient consider options other than euthanasia? If so, which options and if not, why not?

F.   Could anyone else have influenced either the patient or yourself in the decision? If so, how did this manifest itself?

III. SECOND OPINION

A. Did you consult another doctor? If so, please supply all the names, addresses and telephone numbers. If you consulted more than one colleague, please supply all the names, addresses and telephone numbers.

B. What conclusions did the other doctor(s) reach, at least with respect to questions 1F and 1G?

C. Did this doctor/these doctors see the patient? If so, on what date? If not, on what were his/her/their conclusions based?

IV. EUTHANASIA

A. Who performed the euthanasia and how?

B. Did the person concerned obtain information on the method used in advance? If so, where and from whom?

C. Was it reasonable to expect that the administration of the euthanasia-inducing agent in question would result in death?

D. Who was present when euthanasia was performed? Please supply names, addresses and telephone numbers.

Guidelines for the pathologist when euthanasia is reported by an attending physician in the Netherlands

1. The basis of the current procedure for reporting euthanasia is that euthanasia, or assisting a patient to take his/her own life, does not constitute a natural death. The attending physician may therefore not sign a death certificate. The procedure is that the physician notifies the municipal pathologist, who prepares a report for the public prosecutor.

   See the Medical Inspector for Health bulletin "Guidelines for physicians on the regulations relating to burial and cremation" (reprinted September 1987) and section 29t, subsection of the Burial and Cremation Act.

2. Under the procedure in force, a physician who has performed euthanasia must submit to you a full written report giving the reasons for his or her action. The report should cover all the points listed in the enclosed guidelines of 18 December 1990 for the attending physician in reporting euthanasia to the municipal pathologist (ref SB/90/335).

3. Under the provisions of section 29t, subsection 1 of the Burial and Cremation Act, you are to report cases of euthanasia to the public prosecutor by submitting the form referred to in the above-mentioned section of the Act.

4. The following two/three documents must be provided under the item "additional information" under b* of the

above-mentioned form:
a. the report drawn up by the attending physician referred to at 2;
b. if it exists, the living will as referred to II.3;
c. a statement of how you verified the details provided by the attending physician (for example by examining the patient's medical records, inquiring of the doctors consulted).

NB If there are any parts of the attending physician's report which you have been unable to verify, you should make this clear and say why verification was not possible.

Chapter 3

Birth of a law

In 1985 Los Angeles attorneys Robert Risley and Michael White started drafting a law by which patients could lawfully ask physicians to help them to die. The impetus for their action was the recent death of Risley's wife from cancer. She did not ask him or a physician for help to die, but as he cared for her during her last days Risley realized that, given her suffering, she might do so. His legal brain began to turn over the judicial consequences of assisting the death of another for humane reasons. A study of the cases and statutes showed that while it is not a crime to take one's own life, it is a crime to assist that action. Here's a legal ambiguity to start with: It is a crime to assist in doing something that is not a crime!

My first venture into law reform of euthanasia began in 1978 when the London *Evening Standard* asked me to write a Charter for the Legalization of Voluntary Euthanasia (4.24.78). The reason the newspaper chose me was that my book about helping my first wife who had terminal cancer to die, *Jean's Way*, had just been published and was causing a huge controversy. In those days I knew little about the ethics and law of euthanasia. Nevertheless, relying on instincts and common sense, I fashioned a charter which broadly is not unlike the principles we are fighting for today. The fine print remains the problem!

In 1980 I had the idea to start the Hemlock Society. I drew

up its charter, and using the royalties from *Jean's Way* for financing, got the organization going with the help of three colleagues. It was a lonely, uphill battle for the first five years. For the first three years I was the only staff member; then I added one assistant, two years later a second. Hemlock began to be recognized as a responsible, viable organization pleading a cause that had hitherto been taboo in America.

In 1985 Risley and White approached me about helping them develop what they then called *The Humane and Dignified Death Act*. I was the resource for research, history and knowledge of the practical problems which Hemlock members had encountered when practicing self-deliverance. On Hemlock's board at the time was Professor Curt Garbesi, of Loyola Law School, who willingly applied his brilliant mind to help fashion this unique law.

There was no existing statute to build upon. The failed attempts to reform the law in England and in the Netherlands did not involve a detailed law which we knew we had to offer in America if there were to be any chance of success. Many a Saturday morning we congregated in Garbesi's Santa Monica home to debate the latest revisions. White was active in the Beverly Hills Bar Association and kept running the law by their members, receiving some useful criticisms and input. By 1987 the first version of a model law was ready. It was rough at the edges, but it was a start.

It was agreed that Risley would start a new organization dedicated to campaigning for this law to be passed in California and elsewhere. Hemlock's tax status as an educational corporation permitted it to take only a minor role in any political venture. Risley's attempts to interest politicians in the

California legislature were rebuffed completely, so it was decided to try for an initiative, which can be loosely be described as a citizen's referendum. If a majority of votes is secured, the law is passed without referral to the legislature.

As a founding member of the board of Americans Against Human Suffering, it soon became clear to me that this organization was not strong enough to even get the signatures necessary to qualify the initiative, let alone have it passed in an election. Under the strain of trying to gather 400,000 signatures without proper financing, the organization virtually collapsed. Most of the board members jumped ship quickly so that they would not be associated with a disaster.

Risley and I met for lunch at my favorite Mexican restaurant, the Casablanca, on Lincoln Boulevard in Venice, to discuss the crisis. "Shall we drop the whole thing, Derek?" he asked. "We cannot win by any stretch of the imagination." I found myself arguing for the initiative to continue for the sole reason that this unusual law badly needed to go under the spotlight of public opinion.

"You and I know that the campaign is going to fail," I said to Risley. "But let's keep that information to ourselves. Let's have this law debated up and down the state as though it were going to pass. First of all, we shall learn where we are mistaken or lacking. Secondly, it will improve the quality of the debate around the right-to-die if people think it is likely to become law."

So for the next three months Risley, White, Garbesi, I and a few others travelled around California stumping for the *Humane and Dignified Death Act*. It aroused such media attention that an impression grew that it was going to pass into law. Hemlock was host to the 1988 World Euthanasia conference in San Francisco and invited Willie Brown, speaker of the California legislature, to be keynote speaker. It was with a mixture of surprise and delight that I heard him tell the audience, "*The Humane and Dignified Death Act* is going to pass." The next morning's newspapers trumpeted this statement by the state's second most powerful politician.

By the time our allotted five months for gathering 372,000 signatures had expired, we had collected a mere 129,764, all by the volunteer effort of Hemlock supporters. The head of a professional signature gathering firm in Sacramento told me that his staff could have obtained the signatures in three weeks if he had been paid about $300,000. "We tested the Death Act," he told me, "It was a shoo-in." By American political expenditure standards, $300,000 is an insignificant amount, but to us it was the pot of gold at the end of the rainbow. Hemlock had subsidized the campaign to the tune of $195,000, most of which was spent on fund-raising. But the fund-raising style was mawkish, some of it in poor taste, and therefore produced slender results.

Nevertheless, the movement for the right to choose to die gained experience and kudos from the 1988 California campaign. The right-to-life movement boasted in its journals that they had decisively beaten us, but we knew only too well that we had beaten ourselves through weak organization. At that time not enough supporters were willing to step forward to help, physically or financially. A faithful few, particularly in San Diego and the Bay Area of San Francisco, had worked tirelessly. To them goes the credit for making that campaign look credible.

Americans Against Human Suffering learned what it had to do four years later-- have enough money to pay for signature gatherers to ensure qualification for the ballot. Residents of California were exposed to the pros and cons of physician aid-in-dying on a scale never previously experienced. Intellectual elements within the medical profession realized that even if this effort had failed, euthanasia was a coming issue and they had better start formulating their responses to it. In the year following the campaign, the Hemlock Society, benefitting from the heightened visibility, doubled its membership and income.

ALTERATIONS

In drafting terms, many alterations followed. I called a conference under Hemlock's aegis at the Hilton Hotel in Eugene for some 25 people interested in law reform of this subject to debate where we had gone wrong in California and how future laws should be framed. Two days of constructive debate followed and alterations were nearly all agreed upon unanimously.

The 1988 version contained a clause forbidding physician aid-in-dying to pregnant women. The idea had been copied from California's existing Natural Death Act which empowered the Living Will. Inclusion of this clause had offended the ACLU, whose support we needed. It was reckoned that the number of cases of requested death coming from expectant mothers would be minimal, so if it happened, it would be best if a court ruled on the matter. We deleted it.

Under the original version, people could get voluntary euthanasia even if they became incompetent, provided that they had previously given power of attorney to another person while still competent. This aspect of right to die appeals to many people who fear that their final years will be spent in a zombie-like condition after a stroke or from the effects of Alzheimer's disease. So great is their dread that they are willing to have someone else decide the day of their death by a physician's hand.

Americans Against Human Suffering and Washington Citizens for Death With Dignity decided that the public was not yet ready for this second step, because it greatly complicated the legislation. I argued against deletion of what I thought was a crucial clause which attracted many people but the voting went against me. Thus the Washington 1991 and the California 1992 Initiatives to the voter offered physician aid-in-dying only to the patient who could ask for it.

Chapter 4

Ways to change the law

There are four possible ways in America to secure careful and legally protected physician-aided dying for the terminally ill:

1. By having the conviction of a person for assisted suicide dismissed on appeal to an Appellate Court, State Supreme court, or the US Supreme Court.

2. By state legislatures passing revisions of the statutes which currently forbid assistance in suicides.

3. By having guidelines for assistance in dying which are acceptable both to the medical profession and law enforcement authorities.

4. By a direct voters' initiative in the 18 states which allow this method of changing laws.

APPEAL PROCEDURE
Ever since the *Roe v. Wade* case went to the US Supreme Court and the decision gave American women the right to an abortion, many law enforcement authorities have been careful

not to allow certain court cases which have the possibility of causing significant social change to reach the appeal stage. Either they will not prosecute in the first place, or if they do so and fail to get a conviction they will not appeal. Should they lose, a precedent is then set. (It is the decision in appeals to higher courts which can alter the course of law, such as the Cruzan case, not the original decisions or convictions)

Since 1980 several cases have cropped up which would have made excellent potential vehicles for appeals to test the law on assisted suicide. They have come to nothing. While I do not have an inside track on the minds of district and states attorneys, I am left with the suspicion that these lawyers did not want the cases taken farther for strategic reasons.

The man most likely to change the law by this route is Dr. Jack Kevorkian. Attempts to convict him of the murder of some of the individuals whom he helped to commit suicide failed because his state, Michigan, stood alone of all the states in not having a clear law forbidding such actions. But since February, 1993, it does have a hastily prepared law, designed, it seems, just to block his actions. Judging by his published statements, Dr. Kevorkian intends to go on helping hopelessly ill people to die regardless of the new law. If he does, and is convicted, he has the courage, motivation and legal support necessary to mount an appeal that could affect the history of the right-to-die campaign.

Then on May 16, 1993, he helped a 16th person, Ron Masur, dying of cancer, commit suicide but only to the extent of helping him get the carbon monoxide and being present when he chose to inhale it. Immediately, Dr. Kevorkian was arrested on an open charge and bailed. Whether he could be successfully prosecuted remained in considerable doubt.

It has been obvious in the past four years that juries are re-interpreting the laws which forbid assistance in dying. No one wanted to repeat the monstrous sentence of 25 years passed on Roswell Gilbert, aged 75, in Florida in 1986 for shooting his sick and incompetent wife. (He was granted clemency after five years) The subsequent acquittals of Dr. Peter Rosier (Florida), Robert Harper (Michigan), and Richard Bauer (Colorado) were against the weight of evidence. But as the authorities chose not to appeal these decisions, the law was not altered in any way. Nevertheless, it is likely that these acquittals will influence future policies on prosecutions.

LEGISLATIVE ACTION

In early 1992, a handful of bold legislators in Maine, New Hampshire, Iowa, and Michigan introduced into their assemblies laws which would permit assistance in death for the terminally ill. While well-intentioned, these laws were not well drafted, chiefly because the draftspersons had little experience with the subject. The bills in Maine, Iowa and Michigan sought both physician-assisted suicide and active voluntary euthanasia (physician injection). Alone of all its neighbors, the bill in New Hampshire sought only to permit a physician to provide a lethal prescription for a dying person without fear of prosecution, as would happen now. The physician was not required to supervise the administration of the drug.

Although it was sort of compromise, the New Hampshire bill fared no better than the other three. The two legislators who first introduced it told me that resistance from the medical profession was absolute. None of the bills reached the floor of either their respective House of Representatives or Senate and all of the bills have either died in committee or have been

61

shelved. There is talk of some of them being revived.

In 1991 Senator Frank Roberts, Oregon's senior senator, and The Hemlock Society (Oregon) Inc. jointly sponsored *The Death With Dignity Act* before the Oregon legislature. At the committee hearings on the bill two things became obvious. First, most of the legislators were appallingly ignorant of the subject, which indicated that they did not care to research it. Second, the opposition from churches was overwhelming, the only exception being the Unitarians. Again, the bill never got out of committee.

The likelihood of any legislature passing a bill for physician aid-in-dying is remote. Politicians are fearful of speaking out on ethical issues because the religious right would inevitably call for their defeat when they came up for re-election. A reform via the legislature is cheaper than an initiative, but it is not without costs: very few politicians will act unless money is placed in their campaign funds for re-election.

GUIDELINES

One promising approach to securing assistance in dying for the terminally ill could be through the development of a set of guidelines which would be agreed upon by both the medical profession and the law enforcement authorities in every county or state. Helping a patient to die while carefully obeying the agreed guidelines would exempt a physician from prosecution. This is how physician-assisted dying has been practiced in the Netherlands for the last twenty years. As I said earlier, Parliament has now approved the guidelines. The Dutch approach appears to be working well, but it should be borne in mind that the Netherlands is a homogeneous society, with one parliamentary and legal system for the entire country. Politicians are elected by Proportional Representation, making it hard to target an individual, only the party. Judges are elected for life; they cannot be removed unless found to be acting criminally. Such a nation finds it fairly easy to reach a consensus on a thorny subject. Dutch laws on abortion, sex education, prostitution and the use of recreational drugs are extremely liberal.

Whether the guidelines approach in America would work is debatable. With scores of separate law enforcement authorities across the country, can there be agreement on guidelines? With sheriffs, district attorneys, attorneys general and some judges elected by popular vote in often expensive media campaigns, might one of them use a prominent case against a physician to boost the chance of winning? Interpretation of the guidelines could be a matter of individual ethics, which seemed to be the case in 1981 when two California physicians, Dr. Robert Nedjl and Dr. Neil Barber, were charged with the murder of a patient in a persistent vegetative state by disconnecting him from life support equipment. They protested that they had obeyed the guidelines recently agreed upon by the Los Angeles County Bar Association and the Los Angeles County Medical Association for the handling of such cases. The district attorney retorted that these guidelines were meaningless because they lacked legislative approval. The two physicians were twice charged with murder. Each time the case was thrown out. I was following the case at the time, and it seemed to me that the district attorney was motivated by more than his official duty in his dogged pursuit of the physicians. But he was right in saying that the guidelines lacked teeth.

The judge in the final Barber-Nedjl hearing, when dismissing it, noted the absence of legislative guidelines, but it took another ten years before the flaws in the 1976 California Natural Act were rectified. A right-to-life governor vetoed modifications every time they were passed by the legislature.

So we are left with the dilemma that guidelines that do not have the force of law could be flouted by those who do not like them or wish to manipulate a situation. As already remarked, the likelihood of a legislature passing physician aid-in-dying guidelines is not in the foreseeable future. Nevertheless, the drawing up of such guidelines is eminently worthwhile, ready for the day when they could be made official. Such an exercise would also sharpen medical and lay minds to the complexity and sensitivity of the subject.

VOTERS' INITIATIVES

Given the difficulties in persuading enough legislators to pass *The Death With Dignity act*, the near impossibility of getting a significant case to an appeal court, and the legal weaknesses of guidelines, voters' initiatives are probably the best way to break through the barriers to law reform.

Initiative procedures are from one viewpoint true democracy in action. Yet, as seen in Washington and California, even when they appear to have a good chance of winning, they can be frustrated by well-financed opposition campaigns. This is discussed in Chapter 5. As indicated elsewhere in this publication, initiatives are enormously expensive and labor-intensive. No two states have entirely similar initiative procedures. For instance, in California the signatures on the petition calling for a vote must be gathered over five months, while in Oregon two years are allowed. This is not the place to describe and analyze all the different initiative procedures except to say that the rules in Florida are the most constraining.

There also remains the problem of the states that do not have initiative procedures. When several west coast states have passed *The Death With Dignity Act* by initiative this will send a signal to politicians in the other states that it is time to follow suit.

Chapter 5

Do it yourself?

On January 21, 1993, Dr. Jack Kevorkian, the retired pathologist, went to the home of Jack Elmer Miller, aged 53, in Wayne County, Michigan. The two men had previously corresponded and met. Later Dr. Kevorkian departed, leaving behind a cylinder of carbon monoxide attached to a face mask with a tube. Shortly afterwards, Miller put the mask over his nose and mouth and released the clip which had held the tube pinched closed between the gas canister and the face mask. Within minutes Miller was, peacefully and quietly, dead. He no longer suffered from the bone cancer which had kept him in excruciating pain.

This was the ninth person over three years that Kevorkian had helped to die. In any other state but Michigan the man the media has nicknamed "Dr. Death" would almost certainly face prosecution. Michigan's new prohibition on assisted suicides did not come into force until February, 1993. But did Miller need help at all? If he had known where to obtain it, he could have purchased or rented the gas equipment himself. It could have been delivered to his home just like something from a mail order catalog. Undoubtedly Dr. Kevorkian gave Miller some verbal guidance on how the lethal gas was released, but this information could as easily have been conveyed by the customary manufacturer's printed instructions.

Thus the question arises of whether we need physician-assisted dying. Should it be by D.I.Y. (do it yourself)? Do we need to involve the health profession at all? Using my information, many hundreds, perhaps a few thousand, of people all over the world have ended their lives since I first started publishing self-deliverance books. (*Let Me Die Before I Wake: How dying people end their suffering*, 1981 and *Final Exit: Self-deliverance and assisted suicide for the dying* 1991) Desperately ill and pain-wracked people who cannot get a physician to help them, either with an injection or dispensing lethal drugs, resort to using over-the-counter sleep aids coupled with a plastic bag over the head. It is, in fact, the only way the 90-plus Hemlock chapters around the USA have to respond to the constant calls from desperate people who seek their help. Throughout the country numerous Hemlock members who are not physicians have been driven by their compassion to help people to die. They have gone to the homes of the dying with whom they have been communicating and assisted in the death in whatever way was appropriate to the situation-- last-minute instructions on how drugs should be ingested, or guidance on the use of the plastic bag, but mostly providing moral support to the fearful and the lonely. One such man was Steve Blickenstaff, in Santa Barbara. Not long before he dropped dead of a heart attack, Steve said to me, "You know that I go to people's homes to help when I think it's necessary?" I told him that I had some idea of his activities over the years, but that I preferred, for legal reasons, not to hear the details. Steve was a very balanced man, careful and caring, and above all, discreet. As he was not a Hemlock employee, I could not control his actions, nor the many like him. Hemlock staff were forbidden to help people to die under any circumstances except their own family.

Certainly Kevorkian's gas mask technique seems a pleasant and efficient way to go. But there are problems here, too. First, the dilemma of people who, because of paralysis or weakness of their arms, are unable to place the mask on the face and remove the safety clip from a heavy canister. (This is dealt with more fully in Chapter 7, Divide and Rule?)

Second, under existing laws the sellers or renters of the gas equipment, over-the-counter sleep aids or plastic bags could be prosecuted for knowingly assisting a suicide. To be sure of immunity, laws would have to be changed so that the seller could be neither prosecuted nor sued. But such an immunity begs the question: can they sell the equipment to *any* potential suicide? How does the seller differentiate between the terminally ill and the mentally ill? Should a "release" or "waiver" be signed? Moreover, the problem of making the technology for suicide easier is precisely that it will not just be available to the terminally or hopelessly ill, but also for the depressed and the disturbed. The legal and ethical snags grow like a rolling snowball. . . .

Very, very few people in America and Canada are ever charged with assisting a suicide, especially if the dead person had been seriously and irreversibly ill, and violence-- with a gun or a knife-- was not used. Many of those who are charged accept a plea bargain so that their cases never go to trial. But it is the *fear* of prosecution that is the deterrent to physicians and lay people alike. Few people want to risk an expensive court case, embarrassing media attention, and possible conviction. Martyrs like Kevorkian are rare!

So even if the medical profession should finally decide that it will not support any form of euthanasia, the law prohibiting assisted suicide will still have to be modified to permit the act in certain circumstances. How we define those circumstances could be a sensitive matter.

In Norway, Germany, Switzerland and Uruguay, a prosecutor can take into consideration whether the person who was assisted in suicide was terminally ill and if a request had been made for help for humane reasons. If the assister--lay person or physician-- is considered to have acted from honorable intentions to relieve protracted suffering, there is no prosecution. In these countries, motive is the governing factor as to criminality.

Norwegian law stipulates that punishment is not applied when the victim has consented, "or where an actor motivated by mercy takes the life of the hopelessly ill person." Similarly, Uruguayan law punishes no one motivated by compassion to act upon the repeated requests of the victim. Swiss law says prosecutors and judges must consider whether the defendant acted for "noble" reasons. It seems that there are no prosecutions in these four countries because a successful defense could be mounted where terminal illness is involved.

During the debates over legislative change in Washington and California, many physicians said they did not have problems with the idea that a hopelessly ill patient should be able to end his or her life. But, they did not think a physician should be involved either directly or indirectly as a sort of "executioner." Many used the Hippocratic Oath to defend this position; others said it was just not what they were trained or wanted to do as a doctor.

Yet while we slowly pursue the legal changes to permit those doctors who wish to help to be able to do so, many people urgently look for deliverance from their daily suffering. We should be developing legal, simple alternatives that would at least help the majority of those people who are not too weak or disabled to be able to help themselves. Faye Girsh, a clinical and forensic psychologist who is also president of the Hemlock Society of San Diego, comments: "The use of the plastic bag by such people as Bruno Bettelheim is an example of the simple technology whose use was promoted through Hemlock publications, making death painless and easy for countless people who were not likely to choose more violent means." (Letter to the author, February 8, 1993) It appears that the longer the resistance to helping the terminally or hopelessly ill is encountered from physicians, the more likely the possibility that easier and more certain means of suicide will become available to both the hopelessly ill and to those emotionally disturbed individuals who choose to end their lives. Books like *Final Exit* and doctors like Jack Kevorkian are temporary measures. Now is the time for all caring people to come to the aid of the sufferers.

The fundamental reason why most patients do not wish to do it themselves is that they fear a botched attempt. Some individuals have secured lethal drugs, done careful planning, and are supported by loved ones. They feel confident in self-deliverance. But many others-- like Dr. Kevorkian's clients-- either do not have the drugs or moral support, or, more importantly, live in unspeakable dread of waking up, still suffering, when they had intended to be dead.

71

Chapter 6

Doublespeak

There is wide disagreement throughout the movement for the right to choose to die over the best words to use when campaigning publicly for law reform. Not about definitions of words, about which there is little dispute, but whether certain words are unwise to use because they might upset some of the public, *ergo* lose votes. The argument is made that euphemisms are preferable.

Some of the words in question are:

Actual Word	*Euphemism*
Euthanasia	Death with dignity
Voluntary euthanasia	Choice in dying
Assisted suicide	Aid-in-dying
Rational suicide	Self-deliverance
Lethal injection	Medical procedure or physician aid-in-dying

As the reader will probably have noticed, I use both the real words and the euphemisms. The intention is to vary my language and be less repetitive when writing at length on the same subject. But as a rule of thumb I use the word "suicide" when referring to the legality of the act, and "self-deliverance" when referring to it as a personal decision.

The term "self-deliverance" was introduced by me to America in the late 1970s. I had picked it up in Britain from the euthanasia movement there. I also introduced the term "aid-in-dying" which I had come across in the Netherlands. This term was particularly useful when we were drafting the first *Death With Dignity Act*. Because "euthanasia" does not fit well into a statute-- it is too general, too poetic-- "aid-in-dying" is better suited. The problem with "aid-in-dying" is that it can literally mean a whole range of actions, everything from shooting a person to holding their hand in a comforting manner. For the term to be effective we all have to agree on a definition. (See glossary)

I believe in using real words to describe exact situations. Dying and death are too serious subjects for loose language or euphemisms which could lead to misunderstandings causing suffering. My media and lecture-circuit experience indicates that the general public appreciates straight talk in gutsy language rather than pap and jargon of the type used by politicians. Plain language is the secret of Ross Perot's success. To wrap up our purposes in fancy language invites our critics to say, first, that we are trying to change the law in a covert fashion; and, second, that we are ashamed of being frank about what we really want.

But some people feel differently. They argue that the word "euthanasia" has a Nazi connotation. The German program was deliberately called "euthanasia" to hide its true intention, which was an attempt to purify the German race so as to justify Hitler's claim to head "the master race." Unquestionably anything associated with the German barbarities of murdering nearly 100,000 mentally and physically handicapped patients during World War II is extremely negative. The only survey evidence is contained in a poll of 600 registered voters done in Washington state in April, 1991, prior to Initiative 119. This was the question and answers:

What does the term euthanasia mean to you? Does it seem like a positive or negative term to you?

Positive	**20%**
Negative	**18%**
Mercy killing	**12%**
Helping someone to end their life	**9%**
Right to live or die by choice	**8%**
Death not by choice/killing/murder	**8%**
Not sure of exact meaning	**8%**
Ending life	**6%**
Putting someone to sleep	**6%**

If those who had a positive or at least spoke of euthanasia in a kindly way are totaled, it comes to 55 percent acceptance. The negative response (18%) and those who thought it murder (8%) total 26 percent.

Jack Nicholl, a professional political consultant who managed the Proposition 161 campaign in California, is, like his counterpart in Washington State, vehemently against words and terms like "euthanasia," "assisted suicide" or even "Hemlock Society" coming anywhere near the voter. These terms, he argues, offend some people who might otherwise vote for law reform.

John Brooke, a United Church of Christ minister, expresses the same view: "I believe we need to work at changing language on 'aid-in-dying', 'assisted death', etc, using such terms in place of 'assisted suicide', 'killing' etc.-- which will remain pejorative terms for many people because of their common usage/meaning. The word 'euthanasia', although it should be an acceptable term, has been tainted by its association with the Nazi Holocaust, and because 'euthanizing' pets, although a human procedure, is never the result of a 'choice' on the pet's part, thereby leaving the implication that euthanasia is something done to a person sometimes without his or her request.

"The dictionary does not specify request by the patient, therefore 'euthanasia' can be confused with 'mercy killing,'" Brooke continues. "The phrase 'active voluntary euthanasia' attempts to carry the intention that physician assistance must be requested, but 'voluntary' is subject to passive as well as active interpretations; critics may still argue that initiative could come from the doctor or family, not the patient, and still be 'voluntary.' I think it must be clear that initiative and choice are strictly the patient's. I would therefore prefer a phrase such as 'requested physician aid-in-dying.'"

The other side of the coin is whether euphemisms might offend the supporters of change, especially those who notice the contradictions with the real language being used by the medical profession, the media, and, of course, the right to lifers who are constantly twitting the right to die supporters for being "wolves in sheep's clothing."

In the *Hemlock Quarterly* throughout 1988 there was a lively debate in the letters columns over the use of euphemisms. "I think that euphemisms are a form of intellectual dishonesty that we use to shield ourselves from unpleasant truths," wrote the person who kicked off the discussion. "We should and must be honest enough to face the painful reality of death. . . . Only by being intellectually honest about dealing with death, killing and suicide can we maintain a claim to acting morally and ethically," added the writer.

In the following issue of the newsletter a correspondent described how people tittered when she used the phrase "self-deliverance." "It is too jargony. . . I suggest we might use 'mercy suicide' as in 'mercy killing,' thus staying with the existing and accepted words," pleaded the writer.

As the debate heightened, one correspondent said, "Suicide suggests the enraged, the bereft, the love-lorn, the cowardly, and the mentally unbalanced. 'Self-deliverance,' on the other hand, connotes release for the terminally ill, the paralyzed in pain, and the basket case with nothing to look forward to."

But another writer put it this way, "Euphemisms have an important place in our language and often merit respect. . . . Euphemisms can be useful and helpful in calling attention to the attitude and/or the rationale that gives meaning to a specific act. The whole purpose of language is to deal with the complexity of reality. Obviously some euphemisms are dishonest and intentionally misleading, but many others are honest, illuminating and liberating."

The entire correspondence proved only that opinions are deeply divided within the euthanasia movement. What they are in the general public we do not know for certain.

Meanwhile, the medical journals, which of course are not read by the average voter, use the actual words constantly. "Proposed Clinical Criteria for Physician-Assisted Suicide," said a headline in the *New England Journal of Medicine*

(11.5.92). Another headline in the same journal (Vol. 322, #6) read, "Euthanasia-- A Critique." For example, "Assisted Suicide is Not Voluntary Active Euthanasia," read one headline in the *Journal of the American Geriatrics Society* (10.92), while "Maintaining Control in Terminal Illness: Assisted Suicide and Euthanasia" was the headline for an article in *Humane Medicine* (Summer, 1990).

It can only lead to confusion on everybody's part if the proponents of euthanasia and the new law talk in one language and the medical profession in another. Some, like the Reverend Brooke, have even argued that the medical profession must be educated to the alternative words and terms. This could be a fruitless battle.

Like it or not, the public takes its language, particularly in a relatively new field of human activity like euthanasia, from the various forms of news media. Nowadays Jack Kevorkian is labelled "Dr. Death" on television news and that is becoming his popular nickname. He, too, has his pet euphemisms: "medicide" for medically-assisted suicide, and "obitiatrist" for a physician who ends life upon request.

The fear that certain words will hurt their cause is exemplified by the decision of Washington Citizens for Death With Dignity to change its name in 1993 to Citizens for Patient Self-Determination. Explaining why, the president, Dr. Sheldon Biback said, "The past two years have seen two initiatives -- 119 in Washington, and 161 in California, fail at the polls. Both of them were entitled 'Death With Dignity.' This has produced a negative association by the general public between our group and those failed issues, and a reluctance of legislators to deal with us on any issues involving the words 'dying' or 'death.'" (Newsletter, April, 1993). Yet the campaigners in California took an entirely opposite view, altering its name around the same time from "Americans Against Human Suffering" to "Americans for Death With Dignity."

In my 15 years of work in the right to die movement, I have found that the meaning of words to be the most contentious of issues. If we are afraid of the effect of words like "death" and "dying," why is our society so sated with detective fiction about homicide, with true-life murder books, with films and television stories in which death is the solitary plot line? It is curious that our staple diet of entertainment involves death but fear to face up to it in reality.

The right-to-life movement has its euphemisms as well. It calls people who are in a persistent vegetative state because of trauma which has severely damaged their brains "disabled," a term which most of us apply to people with physical or mental handicaps but who still enjoy active lives. People in P.V.S. are bed-ridden, have no cognitive function, and are kept alive by artificial life-support equipment.

Throughout the California campaign in the fall of 1992, the media frequently called Proposition 161 either "the suicide law" or "the euthanasia proposition." Taking all these factors into account, it would be running against the tide not to use actual, truthful words in law reform campaigns.

Chapter 7

Divide and rule?

In the 1970s, the medical profession divided the euthanasia issue into two parts: passive euthanasia (allowing to die) and active euthanasia (helping to die). This was despite the arguments of eminent philosophers like Joseph Fletcher and James Rachels that all acts of euthanasia were essentially the same because an act of omission implied a decision that resulted in death just as much as an act of commission did. I agreed with the two philosophers but never made much of it because if it helped the medical profession deal with the issue as a whole, then the nomenclature was not all that important. If we had to deal with the problem in two parts, then so be it.

But opinion-leaders in the medical profession are now sub-dividing the active euthanasia issue into two parts: assisted suicide (self-deliverance via a physician-supplied prescription drug with the physician perhaps at the deathbed), and active voluntary euthanasia (the physician's injection of lethal drugs into the patient by mutual agreement). Numerous articles and letters are appearing in medical journals suggesting that assisted suicide might be condoned, but not active voluntary euthanasia. We should not let them evade their responsibilities as self-selected healers and caregivers to all of humanity. If an AIDS patient-- today's equivalent of lepers in the eyes of some -- seeks medical help, can an appropriately qualified physician

81

refuse? I believe that one who did decline should be stripped of the license to practice medicine.

For example, putting forth the case for assisted suicide only, three physicians wrote in the *New England Journal of Medicine*, "We support the legalization of (assisted) suicide but not of active euthanasia. We believe this position permits the best balance between a humane response to the request of patients like those described above and the need to protect other vulnerable people."

They acknowledge that this is limiting, though, and some people will be discriminated against. They continued, "We recognize that this exclusion is made at a cost to competent, incurably ill patients who cannot swallow or move and who therefore cannot be helped to die by assisted suicide." These patients should not be abandoned, they pleaded, but given maximum care and pain management. To the credit of the three physicians, they recommended that the physician should be present at the assisted suicide unless the patient specifies otherwise. (Drs. Quill, Cassel, Meier, *NEJM*, 11.5.92)

There are also people in the pro-euthanasia movement who argue for the legalization of assisted suicide now. Quoting the proverb "Half a loaf is better than none," they feel it would benefit a great many people currently suffering, though, of course, not all. Another argument is that experience could be gained about the practicalities and ethics of assisted suicide. There would also be the added benefit that over time physicians would grow comfortable with this compromise procedure and then be ready for active voluntary euthanasia. It would be a step-by-step approach to law reform.

A man who believes in the theory of dividing physician aid-in-dying is Milton D. Heifetz, a neurosurgeon in Los Angeles, who wrote the 1978 landmark book *The Right to Die*. He says, "I strongly believe that when multiple issues are combined in a single measure it is an open invitation to greater controversy. There is a significant difference ethically, legally, logistically and psychologically between granting a physician the right to advise a qualified patient how to die gracefully and the right to commit an act of euthanasia.

"Although I may agree with the validity of both concepts, the latter is fraught with psychological and legal ramifications and its inclusion in a bill permitting assisted suicide appears to be unwise, at least from a tactical point of view. I believe the failure of the Washington (1991) and California (1988) proposals was due to the lack of sharp focus-- the combining of separate issues. It may be much more prudent to approach these problems in a step-wise manner. When society has lived with this concept and begins to realize that life has not been demeaned by such a law, it may then be time to establish a law that would permit acts of euthanasia within set parameters" (*Hemlock Quarterly*, April 1992).

Such a discriminatory solution to a problem is not acceptable. It would mean that if you contracted one terminal disease you would be assured of a peaceful death. If you had the bad luck to contract another illness that left you physically impaired as you were dying, there would be no prospect of escape from suffering.

Consider this scenario: A physician has two patients who are dying. Both ask-- and with justification because of their unrelieved suffering-- for help to die by the use of drugs. The physician is willing to help because a certain respect has grown up between them all during the fight to live, now lost. One patient has advanced bone cancer and will have no trouble lifting the glass of drugs to his or her mouth and swallowing. So the physician supplies the lethal substance and sits with the patient during the dying process. The second patient has ALS (Lou Gehrig's disease) in its advanced stage and cannot move any limbs. Lifting a cup to his own mouth is impossible. The patient is beginning to choke on his spittle and wants to die. But the physician cannot help.

I doubt whether my hypothetical physician could sleep at night knowing that one patient had received a humane and dignified death while the other was lingering on in helpless distress. Elements of the medical profession are looking for an easy way to respond to widespread public dissatisfaction at the modern dying process. Splitting the patients into two camps-- the mobile and the immobile, plus those who cannot swallow-- is not the answer. Apart from the morality, such legislation would bring a flurry of anti-discrimination lawsuits which could soon broaden the law, perhaps in a haphazard manner. Separating the assisted dying issue into two distinct parts is a natural tendency, but there must be one overall solution.

The three physicians who wrote the *New England Journal of Medicine* article sought the compromise solution because they felt that there were too many vulnerable people in America to be able to license physicians to directly end life. They referred specifically to people without medical health insurance, and they presumably also had minorities and illegal immigrants in mind. That America is a land of extremes in poverty and wealth, ignorance and education, good health care and disgraceful lack of it, hardly needs to be repeated. But it has always been so, and regrettably will be for some time to come. These inequities demand other solutions. They should not mean that those who are striving for a more humane societal approach to dying should back off because all of mankind is not equally rich, educated and cared for. If all problems waited for a perfect world before proceeding then no progress would be made at all.

India, which has scores of millions of desperately poor people, has the Society for the Right to Die With Dignity, headquartered in Bombay. Some Westerners ask, "Why do they need such a group when so many die of starvation?" But the poor man dying of cancer in his mud hut is just as deserving of a good death as the rich businessman with the same affliction in his palatial home. "Death hath no dominion," wrote Dylan Thomas.

The best argument for having the new law embrace both assisted suicide and active voluntary euthanasia may come from statistics from the Netherlands. The Remmelink Report (1991), unquestionably the world's most authoritative survey of euthanasia in practice, says that while 1.8% of all deaths in that country each year are by physicians administering lethal drugs, a mere 0.3% are by assisted suicide where the physician intentionally prescribes or supplies them. Where there is a choice, it seems the dying much prefer direct action by the physician. The Dutch do not even discuss the possibility of legalizing assisted suicide only.

The assisted dying law that soon should be agreed upon by the people and the medical profession must be a model of fairness to all, with each side taking its proper share of responsibility. The recommended model law at the back of this book makes distinction of and provision for the two kinds of assisted dying. Those in the American medical profession who take account of public opinion, recognizing the huge, new interest in euthanasia, are giving out a pacifier by their emerging approval of assisted suicide. Some people in the pro-euthanasia movement are sucking on it. But we cannot be selective in which of the dying gets our compassion.

It would be different if a state legislature was offering to bring in a law for assisted suicide only. It has been said that politics is the art of compromise, so I for one would accept the "half a loaf" being offered by politicians. But the harsh truth is that as yet, no majority group of politicians is making any such offer. Therefore when the "death with dignity" movement swings into action with more voters' initiatives it should go for the whole loaf-- assisted suicide *and* active voluntary euthanasia. When the general public fully comprehends the arguments-- as it is starting to-- there will be greater support at the ballot box for a truly fair and humane piece of law reform.

Chapter 8

Doctors who approve

When legalized, the responsibility of assisting suicides will fall onto treating physicians. If one looks at the fact that no medical societies endorsed either the California or Washington State initiatives, it could be assumed that doctors want nothing to do with this. True, some declare that assisted suicide goes against the Hippocratic Oath and therefore must be wrong. Yet in four formal polls and an informal survey it was found that many physicians endorse the idea of their assisting suicides, and almost all agree that a patient should decide on end-of-life treatment or non-treatment. The two voters' initiatives were not endorsed because these groups, it seems, could not agree on the finer details involved in the issues.

A National Hemlock Society poll released in February, 1988, indicates that roughly half of the physicians polled (51% of 588 respondents) would assist patients were voluntary euthanasia to be legalized. Sixty-eight percent, though, thought that the law should be changed to legalize voluntary euthanasia- - it was a choice they respected but not all were willing to practice it. Assuming that the physicians who would practice euthanasia also would support the law being changed, there is a significant number who respect the idea of people taking their lives in a terminal situation, and would perhaps consider aiding patients on a case by case basis. Sixty-two percent said that is sometimes right for physicians to take steps to end death. Of those doctors who had rejected a request for death, nearly 80% indicated that it was chiefly because euthanasia was illegal rather than any fixed attitudes.

A survey taken by the San Francisco Medical Society (reported in *San Francisco Medicine,* May, 1988) also indicates positive support for physician-assisted suicide. Of 676 respondents, 70% agreed that patients should have the option of requesting active euthanasia when faced with incurable terminal illness. When pressed further, 54% indicated that if euthanasia were legalized, it should be the physicians who carry it out. Of those who said that physicians should not be the ones to carry it out (26%), 28 doctors felt that the patient should do it. Another 18 thought a "euthanologist" (similar to Kevorkian's "obitiatrist") should do it.

In this survey, 45% of the doctors said they would practice euthanasia were it legalized. Another 18% were unsure, but were not ruling the possibility out. Again, physicians shared a preference to make decisions on an individual basis.

A larger poll on physician attitudes and practices was taken by the University of Colorado at Denver in May, 1988. Of the 7,095 Colorado physicians who were mailed surveys, 2,218 responded. In this survey, 60% of all doctors who responded had treated patients for whom they thought active euthanasia would be justified were it legal. Of the doctors who had seen these patients, 59% said they would have been willing to administer a lethal drug were it permitted by law. Some of the surveyed physicians (four percent) had assisted patients in stockpiling lethal doses of medication knowing that they would be perhaps used later to commit suicide.

Physician's Management magazine released in 1991 a

survey of 2,000 internists, general practitioners, and family practitioners which showed that over nine percent had deliberately taken clinical actions to end a patient's life. Nearly 45 percent had taken actions that would end a patient's life indirectly, 3.7% had provided information that could be used to end a patient's life, and over 92% had issued DIR orders.

An informal poll by the American Society of Internal Medicine (ASIM) (*The Internist*, March, 1992) uncovers problems that surround polling physicians on this issue. Of the 402 internists who participated in this survey, 80 respondents (roughly 20%) indicated that they had taken deliberate action to end a patient's life. However, they were not asked how many physicians would assist were voluntary euthanasia legalized.

When this poll asked if physicians should refer patients to the organization Choice in Dying, or to my book *Final Exit*, 82 said they did not know enough about the organization and 91 said that they had not read *Final Exit*. Choice in Dying deals largely with the Living Will, a document about which every patient has to be informed, according to the 1991 Patient Self-Determination Act. Why would a doctor not want to make this referral? Clearly a number of physicians are basing decisions on flimsy knowledge of the issue.

Can any poll properly reflect the subtleties of an issue like euthanasia? *The Internist* reported that many respondents said they would need to have more information on the individual cases were they to actually consider whether or not to assist a terminal patient: the polls made the issue too black and white. There are factors that polls cannot cover-- informed consent, patient disposition and attitude, personal convictions and beliefs of all those involved, and other incalculable factors that nevertheless guide daily decisions. Polls indicate a majority of physicians think that patients have the right to make their end of life decisions, with roughly half the doctors convinced that physician-assisted suicide should be legalized. The numbers drop when it comes to physicians who would be willing to assist patients personally, but this would seem to be due partly to physicians only now beginning to develop their ethical positions, and partly to the fact that a good many physicians are in specialties that do not involve dying or death.

In a poll announced in April, 1993, the *Boston Globe* newspaper said it had conducted a survey in cooperation with the Massachussets Medical Association. Of the 837 physicians in the Boston area who treated dying patients and answered the survey, 53 percent said that if it were legal, there were circumstances in which they would honor a terminally ill person's request for "aid in dying" by administering a lethal dose of medicine. Thirty percent said they would not and 15 percent said that they did not know.

It is a favorite ploy of anti-euthanasia physicians to claim that, despite their long experience, they have never been asked for euthanasia. So there was no problem. Yet of the physicians polled in Boston, 21 percent said that they had been asked for a prescription for a lethal drug, while 19 percent said that they had already honored such a request.

On the thorny issue of lethal injections, the Boston poll revealed that 20 percent of physicians had been asked for a lethal injection and 13 percent had already given one. Asked why patients sought euthanasia, the physicians said the single most important factor was the patient's wish not to face increased pain and suffering (71 percent). The next reason was not wanting to be kept on tubes and machines (14%), with a desire not to be a burden on the family (10%).

Perhaps the most fascinating and telling part of the Boston poll was the final question to physicians: What if you found yourself suffering from a terminal illness? Would you be likely to take steps so that you had the option to administer a lethal dose of medication to yourself? The answers were:

Yes, I would	**40%**
No, I would not	**29%**
Don't know	**30%**

Physicians in the Netherlands have been practicing voluntary euthanasia since 1973. In the Remmelink survey commissioned in 1990 by the Dutch government, 405 physicians indicated that 54% had at least once injected lethal doses of medication or provided the means for the patient to overdose. Another 34% said that although they had not yet assisted a terminally ill patient to die, they might in certain situations. Only 11% said they would never practice euthanasia, although all but 3% said they would definitely refer the patient to another doctor.

The Remmelink report estimates that 25,000 patients per year seek some reassurance from their physicians that if their mental and physical suffering becomes unbearable, the doctors will assist them to die. Nine thousand each year are explicit requests for euthanasia. Less than one-third are agreed to, although only 14% are denied for psychiatric reasons. Most of the time doctors work with their patients to find alternatives that make their lives bearable again. Ultimately, as indicated earlier, somewhere between two and three thousand patients in

91

the Netherlands are assisted by their physicians to die each year.

The evidence from all these polls appears to corroborate what a California physician told me: "Physicians in America would not allow themselves to die in the terrible way they put their patients through."

Chapter 9

Lessons from three campaigns

There were many useful details and pointers about how a euthanasia law should be framed learned during the 1991 political campaign in Washington State and the one in California the following year. But none was more important than the lesson that a law which specifically, directly, and constantly affects ordinary people must be written in an easily understood language. The jargon and the eclectic phrases that lawyers use when framing a law may be fine for instances of insurance, legacies, liability and so forth, but they are generally baffling to much of the public.

If the two laws which narrowly failed in each those states had been more clearly written, with the do's and do not's spelled out, they might have had greater success. Some argue that these test runs are necessary to make the public comfortable with the proposed changes and their implications. Certainly more health professionals would have supported reform. While 46 percent of the voters in both states firmly backed the proposed law, a poll taken for CAHS in 1991 indicated another 23% who probably would have voted for an initiative, but shied away because of sheer uncertainty. This nervousness is shown in the polls which demonstrated that about three months before the voting day, some 65-70 percent of the people were in favor. But the more the proposed law was debated during the campaign, the more uncertain some people became. Exit polls showed that younger people were more in favor while older folks-- nearer to death-- were less enthusiastic about the law as offered. With such a crucial issue as life and death, and one's life span running out, who would not be cautious? Nevertheless, some of their fears could have been allayed by a law and accompanying educational literature that clearly addressed some of their concerns.

Earlier, in 1988, the first test run of *The Death With Dignity Act* (at the time called *The Humane and Dignified Death Act*) made in California had exposed vulnerable points in the law. As I have said, that initiative, because of weak organization and lack of money, did not secure enough signatures to qualify. Nevertheless, the accompanying debate was noisy and useful. At the Eugene conference afterwards there was unanimous agreement about improvements to a law to be tried in the future. Unfortunately these were ignored when Washington launched its law reform attempt.

So great was the enthusiasm for the Washington law reform that nearly double the needed 150,001 signatures were gathered. During 1990 the campaign raised $200,000, spent $100,000 of it on gathering the signatures, and went into the battle in 1991 with the remainder in hand. During 1991 the campaign raised $1,657,650 from thousands of donors across the country. Advance polling indicated an easy victory for Initiative 119.

I never liked the law offered in Washington State as Initiative 119. As executive director of the National Hemlock Society at the time, I dutifully gave it administrative backing through staff, equipment and mailing lists, and asked people for donations, but never visited the state to speak publicly for the law. It was too loosely drawn, lacking some of the features for which I had been publicly arguing for years, and was also missing other aspects which were a part of official Hemlock policy agreed upon at the conference in Eugene in the fall of 1988.

Initiative 119 had no special protection for nursing home patients. These people are trapped in extremely vulnerable situations and require extra steps to prevent abuse, especially psychological pressure from family or staff. Requests to die coming from the resident of a nursing home should be authenticated either by an Ombudsman or a review committee.

Several other potential safeguards were never addressed. The mental health profession had requested that psychological evaluations be a part of the 1988 law. There was no mention of this in the 119 initiative. (More on this later when discussing the 1992 California campaign) There was no reporting requirement which would have allowed for annual number and site of euthanasia cases to be monitored. Nor was there any mandatory waiting period between the request to die and its fulfillment. The proposed Washington law made no mention of a restriction on the fees a physician could charge for assisted suicide, gave no reference to maintaining normal medical standards of treatment, and made no suggestion that the family be informed, if possible, of what was about to happen to their loved one.

These failures were compounded by a decision to try to improve the state's advance directives within the same law. This led to confusion by the public as to whether they were being asked to vote upon passive or active euthanasia.

Actually, it was both. The double issue enabled the opposition to charge that active euthanasia was being slipped in under the cover of passive. This criticism was actually supported by some of the proponents' literature which emphasized the reform of the advance directives much more boldly than the physician-assisted dying aspect.

It turned out that the attempt to reform the advance directives was quite pointless because a few months later the Washington State legislature modified and updated this particular aspect of their right-to-die laws. These improvements even had the support of the leaders of the medical profession and the Roman Catholic hierarchy which had both furiously fought and defeated Proposition 119!

The "No on 119" campaign raised a total of $1.9 million and spent the bulk of it in the final month slamming *The Death With Dignity Act* daily on radio and television for having no safeguards worth considering. Additionally, the right-to-lifers used the highly respected former Surgeon General C. Everett Koop to speak on television against Initiative 119, whereas the other side declined to import any big names to counter his undoubted influence on the result. Most of the money they raised came from Catholic institutions in lump sums, while the "Yes on 119" campaign spent huge amounts on printing, postage and telephone costs begging people all over America to contribute. They raised a gross of $1.8 million but may have made a tactical error in spending too much of it on education and not enough ($660,000) on television. Too much of the money may have been spent on campaign staff, offices, literature, and fund raising.

Concerned about association with anything that looked like

assisted suicide or voluntary euthanasia for the dying, the Yes Campaign's television advertisements were plugs for reform of the Living Will. "Opponents of 119 complained that Washington Citizens for Death With Dignity. . . were trying to pull a sleight of hand, that they wanted to slip in the euthanasia option under the cover of more politically acceptable changes," commented a writer in the *Hastings Center Report* (March-April 1992).

Some have blamed two other factors for the defeat in Washington. First, two weeks before polling day Dr. Jack Kevorkian helped two people to die in Michigan. While they were both very sick women and wished to die, neither could be clearly labelled as "terminally ill." They were certainly in an irreversible condition, but because they were not in the category that the proposed initiative was addressing, some people were frightened by this example of how the slippery slope argument might work were euthanasia legalized. Second, a month before voting day, my second wife, from whom I was divorced, committed suicide while the balance of her mind was disturbed. Despite the fact that my former wife and I had not spoken for two years, there was a good deal of negative publicity that sought to blame me for the tragedy.

If Dr. Kevorkian and I were partly responsible for the defeat, then we are both big enough to take our lumps. Bill Clinton in his bid for the Presidency faced fierce accusations of infidelity and draft dodging, yet he stood his ground and repeatedly called the accusations "sad," refusing to be drawn into a mud-slinging match. His ultimate success at the polls showed-- not for the first time-- that the public has had its share of personal tragedies, too, and usually rises above such matters to vote for the fundamental issue. The failure of the 119 campaign can largely be blamed on a flawed law compounded by a marketing strategy that spent its money too soon and in the wrong way in the face of a well-financed opposition campaign that concentrated on last-minute television advertising.

Despite its flaws and negative campaigning against Initiative 119 in Washington, the final count on the November 5, 1991 vote was as follows:

Voting Yes: **701,818**   **(46.4%)**
Voting No: **811,104**   **(53.6%)**

Before the vote was even taken in Washington, the campaign to have *The Death With Dignity Act* passed in California had begun. Some observers, including me, pointed out that supporters of the right-to-die movement were unlikely to be able to come up with another $1.8 million within one year. In fact, to be sure to win, a campaign in the much larger state of California needed to raise $3 million-- a seemingly impossible task given the time constrictions. But during 1991 the issue was "hot," mainly due to Dr. Kevorkian's well-publicized assisted suicides and the remarkable sales success of my book, *Final Exit: Self-deliverance and assisted suicide for the dying.* No one was more astonished than I when the book hit the top of the *New York Times* best seller list and remained there for 18 weeks. In the fall of 1991, it was described as the most talked about book in America.

But it was an illusion to think that because of all this publicity the right-to-die movement could now win a political campaign to reform the law. The religious right was well prepared for another defense of the status quo. From reading all the literature put out at the time by the Catholic Conference of Bishops, the National Right to Life Committee, and smaller groups, it seemed that the euthanasia issue was beginning to assume greater importance for them than the anti-abortion issue. Discouraged by the US Supreme Court's reluctance to strike down *Roe v. Wade*, the election of a pro-choice President, Clinton, and the slow but increasing sale in America of the abortion-inducing drug RU 486, the right to lifers were increasingly turning towards a new issue. Over the years I had noticed the religious right's internal frustration at ever having let abortion rights get a foothold in America, and thinkers within that movement blamed it on their splintered attitudes. Some sections were against abortion in every case, a few thought it was acceptable in cases of rape and incest, others added the proviso of acceptance if a mother's life was in danger. They could not agree on a common policy. The forces that wanted a ban on abortions under any conditions prevailed-- and this perhaps was their biggest mistake. If they had allowed at least some abortions on humanitarian grounds they would have won wider public support.

Few right-to-lifers attack any longer the Living Will or Durable Power of Attorney for Health Care. In the 1970s and 1980s they railed against these documents expressing patients' wishes about end of life treatment and did their best to stop them from being passed into law. Today they claim they support the disconnection of life support systems where a life is being pointlessly prolonged. Some parts of the Roman Catholic Church even issue the Living Wills which their church once vigorously fought.

But assisted suicide and active voluntary euthanasia for

anybody, in any medical condition, is anathema to the religious right. They see it as an affront to their God's authority over their lives; only the deity gives life and only the deity takes it away. Some people see suffering at the time of terminal illness as a necessary preparation for life in heaven. Archbishop Tom Murphy, of Seattle, has spoken of "the redemptive value of human suffering." A Catholic ethicist, Albert Jonsen, has written that "if we abolish terminal misery from our experience, we will foolishly hide an essential measure of our humanity." Armed with such convictions, the religious right intends to use its considerable financial power to stop the pro-euthanasia forces every time law reform is attempted. Intolerant of other people's differing ethical standpoints, they wish the laws of the land to reflect only their beliefs.

The group which had run the failed 1988 Initiative attempt, Americans Against Human Suffering, resurfaced as Californians Against Human Suffering (CAHS), and set about gathering signatures more successfully in 1991-1992. The voter population in California is so huge that it is extremely difficult for any one group to gather the minimum number of 385,000 certified signatures needed to qualify the issue for the ballot over the required five month period. Because so many signatures can be declared invalid because of minor errors-- even the wrong ink color!-- more than 500,000 were needed for the official number to pass scrutiny. Hemlock Society supporters and other people tried their best to get signatures, and the San Diego group led with 37,000, but there was no possibility that enough could be secured by volunteer effort. A professional signature-gathering firm in Sacramento had to be recruited and $286,354 was spent in securing the qualifying signatures. The biggest contributor had been the National

Hemlock Society with $100,000, but all this money was spent on signature gathering. Hemlock could have contributed more money, but, citing the need to help with other campaigns, its board refused to do so. John Foss, a person with AIDS who sits on the Board of CAHS, comments on this: "Just think what would have happened had Hemlock seen the logic of the situation-- that California, being the most populous and one of the most influential states in this country-- with the additional funds to generate proper rebuttal advertising to the Catholic Church's/Hospital's negative campaigning-- we might have easily overcome the narrow 5% loss factor and, at least, we would have had ONE state where this was law. At that point, THEN it would have, and still could, behoove us to spread out to yet another state and start anew with our then-successful effort. One state at a time is the only way that I can see this getting off the launch pad. Of course, at some point, after several states have been conquered, it would be logical to revert to a national agenda, having the backing of a few powerful and influential states on our side."

Thus when the four-month campaign opened in July, 1992, CAHS was broke. (The opposition, of course, had not needed to spend any money up to that point) What little CAHS raised was used to pay a part-time campaign manager and a part-time field worker, together with sundry expenses. There was no fundraising professional employed, and consequently there was not even money enough for flyers, bumper stickers, yard signs or buttons. (Late in the campaign these were provided statewide by the Hemlock Society of San Diego) The millions of people in the vast area of Northern California were covered by one volunteer United Church of Christ minister working out of his home-- a hopeless task despite his heroic efforts. His

101

salary and expenses were paid by My Choice, an unincorporated association formed by Lilian Stevens and a few others, and financed by a legacy from her. He could not have participated on the scale that he did during 1992 without this financial backing. The Initiative's sponsors had no grassroots base, and were looking to the Hemlock chapters in California to provide that. They did not, chiefly because National Hemlock was undecided about backing CAHS. Some of the chapters had educational tax status--and were thus limited in political activity-- and they received no clear activity advice from CAHS. Faye Girsh, president of Hemlock of San Diego, who is a member also of the national board, wrote afterwards, "Because CAHS had decided to go ahead with the Initiative on its own at a time when Hemlock resources and members were involved in Initiative 119 in Washington, the Hemlock board could not fully support the campaign." *(Hemlock Quarterly,* January 1993).

The California right-to-die effort of 1992 was poorly-timed, under-funded, and had sincere but undistinguished leadership. The Yes campaign needed more time to raise money and to create a grassroots base, but the momentum of Washington's Initiative 119, *Final Exit's* fame, the value of being on the ballot in a major election year, and with other factors argued for immediate action. It absorbed a tremendous publicity hammering from a "No on 161" campaign which raised, mostly from Catholic institutions, nearly $3.5 million. The No campaign was financed by an unprecedented practice of raising money through Pastoral letters, homilies and direct collections at weekend Masses. This tactic was widely resented by many Catholics as well as others. For two months a California resident could rarely turn on the radio or television in California without receiving a very professional, highly negative advertisement berating *The Death With Dignity Act*. Thirty eight newspapers came out with arguments against the new law, and advised their readers to vote no. The opposition claimed that 127 organizations-- mostly Catholic, but including many medical groups-- had endorsed their campaign. CAHS boasted 13 endorsements which included the San Francisco and Beverly Hills Bar Associations and the Southern California ACLU, but no medical groups.

Yet despite this overwhelming imbalance, 46 percent of registered voters who went to the polls on November 3, 1992 still favored changing the law:

Voting No: 5,348,947
Voting Yes: 4,562,010

When the campaign proper had opened two months prior to voting day, polling by both camps showed that the affirmative side was clearly destined to win, perhaps by up to 20 percent. The opposition shrewdly decided not to attempt to tell people that physician aid-in-dying was morally wrong, but chose to hammer home a message that this particular law in California was a bad one-- poorly drafted and full of loopholes. "No real safeguards," was their slogan.

This was not true, of course, because the California law contained none of the obvious flaws of the Washington model, and had been re-drafted by Robert Risley and Michael White, the principal authors of the original 1988 Act. But, being lawyers, they fell into the very natural trap of writing "a lawyer's law" and not one suitable for public consumption. To

103

understand where the protections lay in *The Death With Dignity Act*, a person had not only to have fully understood its every line, but also have broad background knowledge of American medical laws. This was because many of the protections which the critics claimed were absent were already enshrined in American law. There would be no reason for most members of the public to have such knowledge. The constant hammering of paid media messages trashing the law were highly effective. It is so much easier to say no to something one does not understand than to take the trouble to put in considerable study of a lengthy legal document in order to obtain a truthful answer. Towards the end of the campaign the opposition trumpeted another damaging argument which had great appeal to the poorly informed: "Even those who believe in euthanasia don't like this law," they proclaimed. To a certain extent this must have been true, of course, but how wide was the dissatisfaction in the proponent's ranks? It was impossible within the time left to assess this.

Another strategic move by the opponents was to keep out of the campaign the name of the National Right to Life Committee which is so closely associated in the public mind with virulent anti-abortion efforts. Similarly, the smaller but more vitriolic Anti-Euthanasia Task Force, which detests even Living Wills, was kept out of the public eye. Supporters from both groups in California represented themselves as being from "Human Life." This is an umbrella pro-life group founded in 1980 and run from Gaithersburg, Maryland, by Father Paul Marx, OSB. Human Life International, to give its full name, is devoted to pursuing anti-choice issues. It opposes sex education, birth control, abortion and euthanasia and sponsors anti-choice groups in small Catholic universities. Proponents of euthanasia in the future need to target and publicize who the key opponents are so that euphemistic and strange names do not confuse the public. There is nothing euphemistic about a new organization to fight euthanasia formed in 1993. The Catholic Campaign for America is also opposed to divorce, abortion, fetal tissue research, artificial insemination, contraception, pornography and homosexuality. It campaigns for better wages for men so that mothers are not obliged to work outside the home.

Those who gave time, effort and money to the California campaign to try to pass *The Death With Dignity Act* were of course disappointed-- although not surprised-- at the defeat. Yet the fight was well worth it. It not only demonstrated that 4.5 million people in one state wanted physician-assisted dying, but it showed the way to produce a much better, nearly flawless, revised version of *The Death With Dignity Act*.

Stephen Jamison, of Northern California Hemlock, has written of Proposition 161: "Although opponents far outspent the proponents, either much more money or much more than money would have been required to win." Jamison's work concentrates on getting health professionals, chiefly physicians, to understand the complexities of euthanasia. He continued, "I found many bioethicists and physicians who were in favor of the principle of physician-assisted dying for the terminally ill but who were opposing 161 because of unanswered questions. They cautiously pointed out that social change of this magnitude requires the best written law." (*Hemlock Quarterly*, January, 1993).

INVOLVING THE MEDIA

The Initiative campaigns in Washington and California suffered badly by attacks in the editorials in which the newspapers give their own views. The No campaigns got the ears of the editorial boards of the newspapers well before the Yes campaigns, and in a very effective manner. This also applied to some television and radio stations. Thus when the Yes campaign people met the editorial decision makers they were confronted by journalists who were well-briefed on the criticisms of *The Death With Dignity Act* and the bulk of the interviews were spent explaining and justifying the law instead of inspiring confidence in it. Consequently, no media of significance endorsed the Act and some advised their readers quite clearly to vote against it. Judging by the final voting figures, not many people were swayed by the media prejudice but in such a close race, every few votes count.

Journalists are not by nature law reformers. They may be keen to root out corruption, correct injustices, and plead for compassion. These topics sell. But altering the established fabric of society-- no matter how rotten-- is not their forte. Offending cardinals, bishops, church leaders and mandarins of the medical establishment on religious and ethical matters is usually farther than most editors wish to go. The best that can be expected is fair and accurate reporting of the debate, and happily there was plenty of this in the recent campaigns.

In light of the experiences in Washington and California, a case can be made for future law reform campaigners to spend their money purely on radio and television advertisements during the month before voting. Educational forums appear to have little effect because they are mostly attended by people

106

with fixed convictions, and leaflets, flyers, pamphlets serve as little more than reminders of voting day.

WHERE THE MONEY CAME FROM

When the dust had settled on the fight, the two sides were obliged to report by the end of 1992 to the California Fair Political Practices Commission on how much they had collected, from whom, and how it was spent.

The "No on 161" Campaign raised a total of $3,510,215 in the short space of the last six months of 1992. It spent all of it and overspent by a further $52,766. The most astonishing part of the fund-raising was that 172,500 people gave $1,489,430 in sums of less than $100, presumably in cash. This was mostly the money collected at Sunday services in Roman Catholic churches, which flowed so rapidly that the campaign had to spend $16,185 on hiring security vehicles from Loomis Armored Inc. to transport it. Another $1,671,667 was raised by gifts of over $100. The California State Council of the Knights of Columbus gave $204,123 and 22 other branches of the Knights contributed sums ranging from $100 to $1,410, making a total of $209,783.

Other Catholic organizations contributed a total of $178,991, including $97,216 in services. The biggest of these donations was $83,529 from the California Association of Catholic Hospitals (in services and supplies), followed by $76,768 from the United States Catholic Conference (cash) and $13,686 (in services and supplies) from the California Catholic Conference. Additional gifts from Catholic organizations ranged from $1,000 from the Immaculate Heart Community in Louisiana to $100 from the Catholic Daughters of America.

The Bishops of Oakland, Stockton, Sacramento, Monterey

(all California) and Spokane (Washington State) kicked in a total of $182,079, while the Archbishop of Los Angeles gave $45,000. For example, the Roman Catholic diocese of Mississippi gave a mere $100 while the archdiocese of Los Angeles gave $116,690. The diocese of Santa Rosa in Northern California donated $26,240. Twenty Catholic churches and religious orders gave total of $54,546, the biggest donations of $20,000 each coming from the Congregation of the Sisters of Charity of Incarnate Work, in Houston, Texas, and The Sisters of St. Joseph of Orange, California. Only four church groups which can be identified as other than Catholic contributed. This was a paltry $1,226.

Medical groups and hospitals contributed an impressive total of $343,300. Twenty of the 31 donors in this group are identifiable as Catholic hospitals. The outstanding donor in this category was $20,000 from Cedars Sinai Hospital in Los Angeles, which is Jewish. Physicians there are known for their views that euthanasia should not be a matter for legislation. "Leave it to our discretion," has been their philosophy, ignoring the criticism that this smacks of their "playing God."

With all this money, collected in the space of only four months, the "No on 161" campaign spent $763,694 advertising on 131 radio and television stations. The remainder went for meetings, speakers, leaflets, mailers and staff time. It is difficult to assess how much money was spent on fund-raising, but considering the huge lump sums which were received it cannot, in many cases, have cost more than the price of a long-distance telephone call.

On the other hand, the "Yes on 161" campaigners raised a grand total of $1,704,607, which was $1,805,608 less than their opponents. It took Americans Against Human Suffering two years to raise this amount, compared to six months. Huge expenditures on fund raising mailers ate up most of the funds and late in 1991 the Proposition 161 campaign was so short of funds that it was obliged to borrow $55,000 from the Security Pacific National Bank in order to keep going. The biggest single expense was $286,354 to a signature-gathering company in Sacramento. A mere $68,870 was spent on radio and television (compared to $763,694 by the opponents).

The largest single donation was $100,000 from the National Hemlock Society. The second biggest donation, $75,097, came from the US Forum and the third, $16,150 from the Funding Exchange. The Voluntary Euthanasia Society of England sent $1,837 and the California group My Choice gave $1,150. Seven individual Hemlock Societies contributed a further $20,585 (San Diego, $17,000; Los Angeles, $1,950; Washington DC, $735; Kansas City, MO, $400; Michigan, $300; North Carolina and Phoenix, $100 each). No churches contributed.

Thousands of individuals across America contributed sums between $10 and $500, the average gift being $35. The biggest individual gift recorded was $5,500 from Lloyd M. Smith, a retired man in Los Angeles, followed by $3,950 from Ms. Elinor Godspeed, a retired person in Washington, Dc, $3,863 from Dr. and Mrs. Allan Johnson, of Palm Springs, and $1,950 from Mr. and Mrs. Edwin R. Morris, retired, in Richmond, VA.

Chapter 10

How to improve the law

The major criticisms of the 1992 California version of *The Death With Dignity Act* were concerned with the waiting period, witnesses and psychological evaluations. In this chapter I deal with those criticisms and a few others.

In my new version of the Act, I divide the requests for physician aid-in-dying into two distinct categories, whereas the previous Acts treated them as one. While I want both to be dealt with under one new law, I define *physician aid-in-dying* in the two following ways:

1. *Physician-assisted suicide*: The provision by a medical doctor of a prescription for lethal drugs to an adult patient who is terminally ill and requests this help;

2. *Active voluntary euthanasia*: The injection by a medical doctor of a lethal substance to a terminally ill patient upon that patient's competent and witnessed request.

WAITING PERIOD

Risley and White succumbed to lawyer's jargon by drafting a sentence which said the request to die must be made by "an enduring request." They defined enduring request as meaning,

"A request for aid-in-dying expressed on more than one occasion." The critics were quick to spot a loophole here. What if the first request was made at 8 a.m. and the second made at 8:01 a.m? Or even a third made at 8:02 a.m? Those brief time intervals did not give time for reflection and assessment by anyone.

Proponents countered that if we tied down patients and physicians to mandatory time schedules and requirements, there could be unnecessary suffering in cases where a timely decision would have brought relief. Is it possible for a law to specify precise details of physician-patient interaction when conditions could vary so? It should not be the purpose of the law to instruct physicians in how to practice medicine. Rather, the law should offer broad guidelines so that doctors are given direction about how to work within the accepted law.

Yet a short waiting period would quiet public misgivings. I recommend a mandatory minimum of 24 hours. Other people recommend longer periods of 48 to 72 hours. To enforce an even longer period could possibly cause unnecessary suffering. Faye Girsh argues, "For some patients who are at home and seriously ill even two trips to the doctor-- or two trips by the doctor to the patient's home-- in a short period of time would create unnecessary inconvenience or suffering. When a doctor has cared for someone during a prolonged illness and a discussion has been made of the options, a waiting period of even 24 hours in unnecessarily cumbersome." Twenty four hours are enough for most investigatory or informational matters to be resolved. It also allows time for the patient to undergo a change of mind. It hardly needs to be said that before the assistance in dying takes place the physician must always ask for a final time, "Are you sure death is what you want?" Only upon a clear, affirmative answer should the service be rendered.

WITNESSES   §1.03 A, B, and C

Under the provisions of Proposition 161, the signing of the Voluntary Directive to Physicians in which the patient asks for an end to life had to be witnessed by two persons not related to the declarant by blood, marriage or adoption. They could not be eligible to gain under any will by the declarant, not be owed money by the declarant, not be a provider of health care to the patient, and not be the owner of a health care facility. That was fine as far as it went, and reflected similar precautions taken in many legal documents.

But during the election campaign the issue arose of whether there should also be witnesses to, first of all, the actual verbal request to the doctor to be given lethal drugs, and secondly, to the actual administration of the potion. Where were the safeguards against a physician, noticing a Directive asking for death in the patient's medical records, recommending strongly in private conversation that the patient would be better off dead? Perhaps the doctor would not be sympathetic to a patient's attitudes, or would not want to admit that he had no further medical options, or that he could not find a colleague to take over while he went on holiday, or treat if the patient's health insurance were to run out.

A case can be made for drafting a law which says that, in addition to the signed Directive, the verbal request to die must be made in the presence of two witnesses who should be informed at the time that they might later be asked to attest to this request. For practical reasons, these witnesses could include family or hospital staff, but not physicians. Even more

113

important would be witnesses on the scene at the actual time point when the lethal drugs were administered to the patient so that the final question by the physician, and its answer, could be heard and later attested to. This particular safeguard should have great appeal to the medical profession.

But there can be snags to even good ideas. When considering the idea of witnesses being physically present, the question of possibly breaching confidentiality between physician and patient has to be taken into account. A patient's right to privacy in decision-making could be hurt if there must be witnesses required at every stage. If you do not want other people, particularly strangers, at your deathbed, should the law force you to put up with them? Or is that an infringement of personal liberty worth tolerating in order to avoid further pain and suffering? Robert Risley says of this, "I strongly resist the requirement of a witness present at the time of death, except upon the patient's request. Death is a private matter now for everyone which I believe is protected by the state and federal Constitution. If anyone is to be present at the time of death, it has to be at the patient's request. It should be a family member, dear friend, minister, priest, or other clergy, for the 45% of the population who are religious."

Undoubtedly we should respect the rights of a patient who wishes to die in private, with only the doctor present. My model law includes a provision that if the patient requested the witnesses to leave the room after they had heard the exchange, that could be permitted, and the patient would die privately.

THE WRITTEN DIRECTIVE   §1.28

What if a physician is presented with a Directive which was signed and witnessed 30 years earlier? It would still be legally valid but the medical staff could justifiably question whether the document truly represented the patient's thinking now. It must be recognized that the Directive is merely preparing the way for the two verbal requests (witnessed by two people being present) which constitute the true test of eligibility for voluntary euthanasia: Does the patient have the mental capacity to decide? Both the Directive and the verbal requests are invalidated if the patient is declared unable to make an informed decision. The Directive not only indicates the patient's long term thinking, but is part of the documentary evidence which is essential to the whole procedure to protect against haste and abuse. Charles Baron, professor of law at Boston College, comments, "Our main focus should be upon the requests made when death is impending. It is these later requests that we should surround with whatever procedural protections we want to require. It is at the point when the requests are made that we want to make sure that the patient is competent, free of duress or temporary influences, and informed as to all alternatives" (Letter to the author, February 19, 1993).

TERMINAL CONDITION   §1.02 j

The most troublesome phrase, in public relations terms, of the 1988 and 1992 versions of *The Death With Dignity Act* were the words in the Directive which said that the patient did "voluntarily make known my desire that my life shall be ended in a painless, humane, and dignified manner when I have a terminal condition or illness, certified to be terminal by two physicians, and they determine that my death will occur within six months."

In their definitions, Risley and White said that "terminal

115

condition" means an incurable or irreversible condition which will, in the opinion of two certifying physicians exercising reasonable medical judgment, result in death within six months."

Some people erroneously interpreted this to mean that the patient must wait six months before they could be helped to die. Others concentrated their criticism on the impossibility of a physician being absolutely sure that a patient would die within this set period. Why six months and not three or nine months? Defenders of the proposed law pointed to the words in the definitions which speak of "opinion" and "reasonable medical judgment" while agreeing that there was probably no such thing as a medical certainty. But this answer did not help.

The purpose of these words, and the spirit behind them, in the proposed law was that only people in the last desperate stages of their illness could take advantage of it. It sent a message to others with early-stage terminal illnesses that they ought to use the best available medical care to fight for their lives, and perhaps usefully prolong them. The six month clause was intended to counter the criticisms that with *The Death With Dignity Act* in place many people would insist on having their lives ended immediately when they were told that they had cancer or AIDS.

The time period of six months was selected because similar periods are frequently quoted in other medical laws, but principally because the hospice movement requires that a person must be likely to die within six months before they can avail themselves of palliative care. It has to be considered whether phrasing such as the patient being in an "incurable and irreversible condition causing prolonged, unbearable mental and physical suffering" would be sufficient justification to ask to be helped to die. Elsewhere in the rewritten law there is stress on alternatives and pain control.

John Brooke states, "Taking out any specified length of time will lead to even greater opposition than faced Proposition 119 or 161. It in effect opens the law to use by <u>chronically</u>, not just <u>terminally</u> ill patients as usually defined (e.g. Alzheimers, or any progressive, degenerative disease for which there is no known cure). This may be desirable to many of us, but will greatly complicate winning general approval. I believe that a separate effort should be made to deal with chronically ill patients. This Act is not the place for that effort. Opponents will attack the imprecision of any terminal illness diagnosis, as they did effectively in their TV ads. We must highlight the patient's awareness of this factor, as spelled out in the directive, and make a strong case, based on statements of terminally ill people, that most patients will not opt for physician aid-in-dying except as a last resort."

The danger of keeping a time limit is that a lawsuit could be brought by a person who was undergoing considerable and hopeless physical suffering, but who could not positively be medically defined as imminently dying. This person could argue that he was being discriminated against by *The Death With Dignity Act*. In fact, such cases were threatened in California if it were to have passed , and undoubtedly they had some merit. Robert Risley comments, "The six months time limit should be retained. Two physicians could readily agree that a victim with HIV infection was and is irreversible, incurable, and only palliative treatments are available following the onset of symptoms. Yet that patient could well live five to

117

ten years following the diagnosis. We do not want a law which would permit HIV positive people to end their lives when there is no symptomatology. This same argument applies to a number of other areas. The criticism of such a law without a time limit would be far worse than the criticism with one. If we use the word 'imminent' or 'immediate' or 'very near death,' we will in effect preclude those patients in serious pain from the benefits of the statute because they could not opt out until they were near dead anyway. Thus, they could not avoid the horrible agonies of the last three or four months of life which is the primary purpose of this legislation. Thus, I feel very strongly that the six months provision, although not perfect, must be retained. Moreover, MediCare uses this cutoff date for purpose of funding and for purposes of defining the terminal condition. The six months provision is one used in medical practice today."

Despite the easy ammunition it gives to opponents, it is preferable to retain the "likely to die within six months" clause.

FAMILY NOTIFICATION   §1.14

The Directive within the 1992 Act contains the words signed by the patient, "I will endeavor to inform my family of this Directive, and my intention to request the aid of my physician to help me to die when I am in a terminal condition, and take those opinions into consideration. But the final decision remains mine. I acknowledge that it is solely my responsibility to inform my family of my intentions."

The critics, as part of their "family values" stance, claimed that it should be mandatory that the family be informed. "You could be killed without your family knowing," they cried.

It has always been the hallmark of right-to-life zealots that

118

they claim to believe that everybody has both a full complement of family and they all love each other and have their best interests at heart. True, there are many such family units, and it is ideal that the family be aware of and perhaps involved in the euthanasia. Not only would I strongly recommend it, but common sense indicates that in the majority of cases the family would know what was going on anyway.

There are also people who have little or no family, or they are not on good terms with their kith and kin. There are persons with AIDS who have been disowned by their families. I have heard of persons with AIDS who have firmly requested nonheroic measures or who designated their lovers as their Attorneys in Fact-- only to be contradicted in their wishes by family members in denial. To mandate that everybody must tell their family would be an intrusion into the rights of personal liberty and privacy which no thinking person would countenance. This is one criticism that we should ignore while at the same time strengthening the recommendation for family involvement as I have done in the model uniform law.

PSYCHOLOGICAL EVALUATIONS   §1.15

The first drafts of the Act back in 1987 did not contain any reference to assessing the mental health of a patient who was requesting death. At the request of several psychiatrists, a clause was inserted because the drafters agreed that this was a useful suggestion. They added:

"Consultations. An attending physician who is requested to give aid-in-dying may request a psychiatric or psychological consultation if that physician has any concern about the patient's competence, with the consent of a qualified patient."

A protest went up from the right to lifers that there was no

119

scope within the Act for psychological assessment until it was pointed out to them that it did exist in the law. Then, with their usual total disregard for personal liberties, they said that the wording was pointless unless the tests and counselling were mandatory! If the critics had their way and removed the words "with the consent of a qualified patient" from the mental health evaluation request, a successful *Death With Dignity Act* would unquestionably be struck down by the US Supreme Court as an infringement of well-established liberties. It was one of the worst features of Soviet Russia that they forced dissidents into psychiatric wards and had them committed permanently. Apparently the right-to-lifers in America want similar draconian powers.

In this instance, as with family notification, a measure of common sense should prevail in interpreting the law. A patient asking to die who then refused the physician's suggestion that it would be preferable if a mental health expert were involved would be harming his plea. I think most patients in this situation would respond, "Send the shrink around. He'll see that I'm as sane as you!" The patient may, or may not, be right, of course. To an uncooperative patient, the physician would be entitled to ask that unless the patient was willing to help him, then why should he help the patient? There are some human affairs for which we do not need to legislate!

There is a legitimate concern that a patient's competency might be compromised by depression brought on by the pain and suffering of the illness and the prospect of death. It is justifiably argued that many depressions would respond to treatment and therefore life could be prolonged. Voluntary evaluation would take care of this. However, it should be noted that the right of any patient-- terminal or not-- to refuse unwanted medical treatment-- as upheld by the Supreme Court in the Cruzan case-- is not contingent on psychological clearance. Nor is there any concern shown by the psychiatric profession or right to life communities about possible depression in the hundreds of cases annually of death brought about by requested disconnections of life-support systems.

A physician who was proposing to help a patient die would be breaking existing law if he or she did not counsel the patient about alternatives. Any change in this area of *The Death With Dignity Act* should be resisted while at the same time finding ways to educate the public about the value of existing informed consent laws. Again, we could strengthen the advisory wording in the model law by saying that if a patient refused psychological assessment this could be grounds for a physician's refusal to cooperate.

PAIN CONTROL AND ALTERNATIVES §1.04

We must respond to the spurious claim by hospice and others that all pain can be controlled, while at the same time recognizing that much of it can. In an articles published in the *New England Journal of Medicine* by Drs. Quill, Cassel, and Meier (November 5, 1992) the important point is made that, "In fact, there is no empirical evidence that all physical suffering associated with incurable illness can be effectively relieved."

It remains true that if a dying patients are "snowed" with narcotics and put into a sleep from which they will not wake, then there is no physical pain. Some people desire that type of dying, but others do not. The right-to-die movement is wholeheartedly behind good pain control and the hospice movement. There should be as little euthanasia as possible. But pain control is not the only relevant issue for some patients in choosing physician aid-in-dying. Even if all pain could be controlled, some patients would still experience "suffering" or a severely diminished "quality of life." This could lead them to seek physician-assisted death. It is important that we allow ample latitude for terminally ill patients, if mentally competent, to judge for themselves when it is no longer tolerable to continue to live. Wording should be inserted into a revised law which makes it clear that, where appropriate, all acceptable measures of pain and symptom control have been exhausted, and that all medical alternatives acceptable to the patient have been tried.

DOCUMENTATION AND REPORTING   §1.23

The reporting provisions of the 1992 Act need careful examination. It said, "Hospitals and other health providers who carry out the Directive of a qualified patient shall keep a record of the number of these cases, and report annually to the State Department of Health Services the patient's age, type of illness, and the date the Directive was carried out. In all cases, the identity of the patient shall be strictly confidential and shall not be reported."

In a perfect world, this would suffice. But it is obvious that especially in the first few years after enactment, this law is going to be ruthlessly examined under a microscope. Critics will pounce upon every perceived weakness or abuse, seeking evidence to have the law repealed. Such attacks can only be dealt with by close examination of the facts of every individual case to test the merits of the criticism. As the price we have to pay for the blessing of available euthanasia, we must sacrifice confidentiality as long as any necessary revelation is *after* death.

I would retain the wording of the 1992 Act because what is most needed is a close watch on how much euthanasia is happening, and who is most active in performing it. I would, however, add the following:

"In the event of a complaint about the conduct of a specific case of aid-in-dying, all pertinent Directives, Advance Directives, medical records, witness statements, and any other evidence must be immediately made available to a review body as appointed by the State Attorney General." (It should be noted that if the police are concerned about an assisted death they already have the power to investigate, and if necessary, the DA could prosecute under the criminal sanctions contained in *The Death With Dignity Act*)

VIDEO OR AUDIO TAPED WISHES

Increasingly, law enforcement officers are using video and audio tapes as evidence before courts so that they cannot be accused of taking biased or edited statements to secure convictions. Most courts now accept such evidence providing it is properly presented, with clear statements as to when and where the recording was made, and by whom and for what purpose. Dr. Kevorkian has shrewdly had his clients make short tape recordings about their desires to be assisted in their suicides. Undoubtedly this has helped him deal with the district attorneys who were anxious to prosecute and the public who wondered about the voluntariness of what he was doing.

In future versions of *The Death With Dignity Act* there could be a provision for the taping of a patient's request to die, and the physician's response. Certainly a video tape of the encounter would add weight in a subsequent dispute, or court case, about the course of events prior to the death. Videos are preferably to audio tapes because verification of the individuals is more obvious. But an audio tape is a good second best if filming is impossible.

I do not think it necessary to include provisions about taping in the Act. But if people wish to add a video or audio tape to their signed directives, then that is a wise safeguard.

DEATH BY COMMITTEE?

Any attempt to force dying people who want relief from their terminal suffering to put their case before a court of law, an ethics committee, or some sort of tribunal of their peers, should be resisted. Once the choice in dying is removed from the individual patient, he or she becomes an instrument of other peoples' values. This would be an abdication of individual freedom. Only the individual can make a quality of life decision concerning their feelings and values.

For instance, Senate Bill 1301 introduced into the Texas legislature in the spring of 1993 by Senator Gonzalo Barrientos would make physician-assisted suicide lawful for terminally ill persons, but stipulated that the patient must first petition the Probate Court for permission. The patient either had to attend court or, if too ill, could be visited by an attorney who would report the facts back to the judge. Within seven days the judge could decide to issue a certificate giving permission to physicians to end the patient's life. It was required that the physician, who could decline to help, should have two adult witnesses present at the deathbed.

Although commendable in some ways, this law in practice

would be difficult to operate. The dying patient would have to get an attorney to help approach the Probate Court in an official manner. Perhaps the patient could not afford or find an attorney? The strain of the dying process upon both the patient and the family are enough without adding expensive legal battles. While it is true that the court only gives permission-- it does not instruct-- a physician to assist the death, it smacks of courts practicing medicine. This is anathema to the medical profession. More fundamentally, the proposed law infringes the liberty of an individual to choose the manner, timing, and means of his or her own death. Judges have biases like everyone else, and one belonging to the religious right, or an Orthodox Jew, might not have a lot of sympathy with the petitioner.

At the time of writing, this Bill-- along with about ten others in America which were either for or against physician-assisted suicide-- lay bogged down in legislative committees.

PHYSICIAN QUALIFICATIONS §1.02 a

A spurious part of the campaigns against *The Death With Dignity Act* in both Washington and California was the allegation that "Any doctor could end your life. Even your eye doctor could kill you!" The short answer to that, of course, was that the proposed law spoke always of the "treating physician." It defined him or her as follows:

"'Attending physician' means the physician selected by, or assigned to, the patient who has primary responsibility for the treatment and care of the patient."

Eye doctors not only do not choose to treat patients for cancer, heart complaints or other bodily physical conditions, nor are they permitted to by hospitals or health insurance companies. Moreover, an eye doctor treating somebody for a bodily ailment would risk being called a "quack" and also be highly vulnerable to an expensive malpractice lawsuit. How many patients with cancer would choose to turn to an eye doctor for relief even if the hospital or insurance company permitted it? The wording of the 1992 law should be changed by using a term to more accurately pin down which specialty or specialties of medicine could end a patient's life.

Some have argued that it would be preferable to have one of the two physicians involved be a specialist in the disease from which the patient was suffering. Ideally, yes, but the trouble of getting the specialty to the deathbed on time, and the added expense (perhaps $750) of having the expert opinion, could cause problems.

It would be preferable to add the following to avoid opthamologists, podiatrists, or pathologists from terminating a patient's life: "Only medical clinicians (as opposed to pathologists who do not treat patients) who in their ordinary course of practice treat dying patients are permitted to assist in a patient's death. Medical subspecialties such as opthamologists and podiatrists are not permitted to assist their patients to die."

THE SECOND OPINION FROM A BUDDY   §1.13

The Death With Dignity Act correctly ordered that a second physician must be asked to agree that the patient is terminal and close to death. But there are many practical difficulties in the way the Act restricted who shall constitute the second opinion. The Act said:

"Independent physicians. The certifying physicians shall

not be partners or shareholders in the same medical practice."
This would work in private hospitals because all physicians are independent and not employed by the hospital. But patients who are enrolled in a large group practice, or health maintenance organization, such as Kaiser Permanente, could have trouble finding a physician who is not on the payroll. Health insurance policies often restrict patients to physicians who are on their approved lists. If the patient was being treated in a large hospital run by an HMO it might be impossible to find an independent physician. This would not be a problem in a public or private hospital where physicians work independently.

This clause was inserted at the suggestion of some physicians who complained that it would be too easy, either through loyalty or pressure, for the second opinion to be obtained casually from physicians who were close to each other, fiscally or by sharing the same office space. More important are the practical problems facing the patient who is in a crisis, and we should rely on the second physician being aware of the serious responsibility of his approval being given.

SUICIDE CLINICS §1.12 and §1.26
Some people have the fear that once *The Death With Dignity Act* is passed, unscrupulous entrepreneurs will establish centers where people can go to be assisted in their suicides. In the short story "Welcome to the Monkey House," Kurt Vonnegut popularized the futuristic idea of "Ethical Suicide Parlors" where people could go to obtain an easy death. The motive for these fictional parlors was to cull an excessive population a hundred years from now, not provide relief from

pain and suffering.

Dr. Jack Kevorkian has written a blueprint for establishing suicide clinics throughout his state, Michigan. It is a highly bureaucratic structure wherein the dying patient must be seen by no less than five medical persons before permission could be granted. It will never happen. It does not need to happen. With a tightly-drawn law to guide them, and a suspicious public watching their every move, physicians who want to help certain patients to die by request will do so circumspectly. The act should be encouraged to be semi-private, with only close family and treating medical professionals involved, to preserve the dignity which the occasion deserves. The example of the hundreds of abortion clinics which are operating legally and ethically is a good one.

But will there be maverick physicians setting up suicide clinics trying to make a fast buck? *The Death With Dignity Act* had this to say: "Fees. Fees, if any for administering aid-in-dying shall be fair and reasonable." It is hard to imagine any fee greater than $200 for the time a physician needs to be with the patient and the costs of the small amount of lethal drugs needed to end the patient's life. From the evidence developed in the Netherlands where only two percent of all deaths are aided by physicians, euthanasia specialists will have a lean time. There are only so many people dying at any given time in any community; the best advertising in the world will not persuade more people to die! In America a physician is free, within certain laws and licenses, to practice where and how he or she wishes, and could conceivably open a suicide clinic. But the legal difficulties, the low financial return, and the moral disapproval which would be engendered in the community, would stop a doctor from starting a business of this type. Should the law ban any fee being charged, relying instead on the physician's beneficence, as an additional safeguard? I think not. Everybody is entitled to remuneration for his work and euthanasia practitioners should not be excepted.

For those who still fear euthanasia entrepreneurs I have inserted a clause in the act (§1.26) barring the establishment of suicide or euthanasia clinics in the state.

RESIDENCY

Desperate for every stick with which to beat *The Death With Dignity Act*, the religious right raised the specter of Washington and California becoming meccas for dying people who knew they could get assisted suicide when ready. This is not an uncommon complaint. It was mentioned again at New Hampshire's hearings on physician-assisted suicide in February, 1993. If it happened it would throw an extra burden on both private and public hospital facilities and health insurance.

"The local taxpayers would be stuck with the bill when people came from other states and other countries to take advantage. Indigent people who come to California and then change their minds about physician-assisted suicide would have to be cared for at taxpayer expense," said a flyer from the "No on 161" campaign.

This has not happened in the Netherlands. The medical profession there is united in saying "No visitors" and I have yet to hear of a break in the ranks. The first state in America to pass *The Death With Dignity Act* should make the same public statement and advise people to pressure their own politicians to reform local laws. Once one state achieves law reform there will be a "domino effect" in the others.

Without doubt a few desperate people will seek help by rushing to the first state to pass the law. Are we so uncaring that we will forbid this? The number of supplicants would probably be negligible. Most dying people are either not strong enough to travel and/or want to die at home comforted by their loved ones. The complications of transferring medical records, health insurance coverage, and finding a willing doctor are additional barriers. Most doctors would insist on time to study the cases brought to them by hitherto unknown patients. On the other hand, well-off people seeking help would bring money into the state and be an economic asset. The religious right chose to ignore the possible benefits.

From my experience, some physicians will help some patients to die, but no physician will help just anybody to die, not even Jack Kevorkian, who is most selective in his clients. It is interesting to note that to date only four of his sixteen clients have been from out of state.

CONCLUSIONS

Before there is another vote on *The Death With Dignity Act*, it needs to be scrupulously fine-tuned to meet sensible criticisms. Everything possible must be included to prevent abuse while giving physicians the confidence to use the law in appropriate cases. It would be a serious mistake to think that society could legislate cleverly enough to embrace all the complexities and variations to which human nature and medical practice are prone. A solution to this would be a solidly organized and well-financed publicity campaign to respond immediately to misleading allegations, thus minimizing confusion and allowing voters to address the true issue. To a certain extent, the law has to be painted with a broad brush. After a couple of years of experience we might need to touch up a few points-- a customary practice in the rule of law. Nearly all of America's 47 states with Living Wills have had to modify them.

If a thousand protections were built in, the religious right would still never accept *The Death With Dignity Act* because it offends their ethics. But the opposition can be thwarted with a more tightly written law based on the experience of three campaigns. More importantly, it will gain increased support of the medical profession.

Two documents must accompany the next attempts to pass *The Death With Dignity Act* into law:

1. A set of legal and ethical guidelines for physicians and other health professionals to takc into consideration. The Dutch guidelines in Chapter 2 can be the foundation upon which American guidelines can be constructed.

2. An explanatory booklet for public consumption showing how protections against abuse, both by health professionals and family members, are enshrined in this and other laws.

As soon as the law takes effect the pro-euthanasia movement should establish a permanent Task Force on Physician-Assisted Dying to oversee and monitor the working of the new rules. At minimum it should comprise one health professional, one attorney and a social scientist/statistician.

131

The work of the Task Force would be:

1. To answer queries from the public, physicians and hospitals about the detailed application of the law;
2. To educate health professionals and the public about the broad purpose and limitations of the law;
3. To keep extensive records of the extent, manner and site of known euthanasia cases;
4. To work with the courts if and when the Act is legally challenged.

Self-policing *The Death With Dignity Act* will make a smoother introduction, and ensure that it is only used by those for whom it is intended. It is a matter of regret that nobody knows how well, or how badly, the Living Wills operating across America actually work in applying passive euthanasia because mechanisms were never put into place to monitor their use.

A uniform model Death With Dignity Act

§1.0 TITLE

This title shall be known and may be cited as The Death With Dignity Act.

§1.01 DECLARATION OF PURPOSE

The people of _____ State declare:

The purpose of this Act is to provide mentally competent terminally ill adults the legal right to voluntarily request and receive physician aid-in-dying. The Act protects physicians who voluntarily comply with the request and provides safeguards against abuse.

In recognition of the dignity which patients have a right to expect, the State of _____ recognizes the right of mentally competent terminally ill adults 1) to make a voluntary revocable written Directive instructing their physician to administer a medical procedure to end their life in a painless, humane and dignified manner. 2) Alternatively, a patient may request a prescription for lethal drugs and the doctor may supply this document without fear of prosecution.

The Act is voluntary. Accordingly, no one shall be required to take advantage of this legal right or to participate if they are religiously, morally or ethically opposed.

§1.02 DEFINITIONS

The following definitions shall govern the construction of this title:

(a) "Attending physician" means the physician selected by, or assigned to, the patient who has primary responsibility for the treatment and care of the patient. Only medical clinicians who in their ordinary course of practice treat dying patients are permitted to assist in a patient's death. Medical subspecialties such as opthamologists or podiatrists are not permitted to assist their patients to die.

(b) "Directive" means a revocable written document voluntarily executed by the declarant in accordance with the requirements of §1.03 in substantially the form set forth in §1.28.

(c) "Declarant" means a person who executes a Directive, in accordance with this title.

(d) "Life-sustaining procedure" means any medical procedure or intervention which utilizes mechanical or other artificial means to sustain, restore, or supplant a vital function, including nourishment and hydration which, when applied to a qualified patient would serve only to prolong artificially the moment of death. "Life-sustaining procedure" shall not include the administration of medication or the performance of any medical procedure deemed necessary to alleviate pain or reverse any condition.

(e) "Physician" means a physician and surgeon licensed by the Medical Board of _____ State.

(f) "Health care provider" and "Health care professional" mean a person or facility or employee of a health care facility licensed, certified, or otherwise authorized by the law of this state to administer health care in the ordinary course of business or practice of a profession.

(g) "Community care facility" means a community care facility as defined in Section _____ of the Health and Safety Code.

(h) "Qualified patient" means a mentally competent adult patient who has voluntarily executed a currently valid revocable Directive as defined in this section, who has been diagnosed and certified in writing by two physicians to be afflicted with a terminal condition, and who because of pain and suffering together with loss of normal quality of life has expressed an enduring request for active voluntary euthanasia. One of said physicians shall be the attending physician as defined in subsection (a). Both physicians shall have personally examined the patient.

(i) "Enduring request" means a request for humane, medically assisted death, expressed on more than one occasion with a waiting period of a minimum of twenty four hours between the first and the final request.

(j) "Terminal condition" means an incurable or irreversible condition which will, in the opinion of two certifying physicians exercising reasonable medical judgment, result in death within six months. One of said physicians shall be the attending physician as defined in subsection (a).

135

(k) "Aid-in-dying" means a medical procedure, or action, that will terminate the life of the qualified patient in a painless, humane and dignified manner whether administered by the physician at the patient's choice or direction or whether the physician provides means to the patient for self-administration.

§1.03A WITNESSED DIRECTIVE FOR ACTIVE VOLUNTARY EUTHANASIA

A mentally competent adult individual may at any time voluntarily execute a revocable Directive governing the administration of active voluntary euthanasia. The Directive shall be signed by the declarant and witnessed by two adults who at the time of witnessing, meet the following requirements:

(a) Are not related to the declarant by blood or marriage, or adoption;

(b) Are not entitled to any portion of the estate of the declarant upon his/her death under any will of the declarant or codicil thereto then existing or, at the time of the Directive, by operation of law then existing;

(c) Have no creditor's claim against the declarant, or anticipate making such a claim against any portion of the estate of the declarant upon his or her death.

(d) Are not the attending physician, an employee of the attending physician, a health care provider, or an employee of a health care provider. The Directive shall be substantially in the form contained in §1.28.

§1.03B WITNESSED DIRECTIVE FOR PHYSICIAN-ASSISTED SUICIDE

A mentally competent adult individual who is terminally ill may request a physician for a prescription for lethal drugs by signing the Directive which shall be witnessed.

§1.03C WITNESSED REQUESTS

If the patient has chosen active voluntary euthanasia, both the first verbal request for death and the final request shall each time be made in the presence of two witnesses who are not physicians but who would later testify if required to what they saw and heard. The witnesses need not be present at the moment of death if the patient requests privacy.

§1.04 PAIN CONTROL AND ALTERNATIVES

No request for either form of physician aid-in-dying shall be acceded to unless all reasonable pain control techniques and other alternatives to dying have been offered to the patient and have been declined as unacceptable.

§1.05 SKILLED NURSING FACILITIES

A Directive requesting active voluntary euthanasia shall have no force or effect if the declarant is a patient in a skilled nursing facility as defined in the Health and Safety Code an intermediate care facility or community care facility at the time the Directive is executed unless one of the two witnesses to the Directive is a Patient Advocate or Ombudsman designated for this purpose pursuant to any other applicable provision of law. The Patient Advocate or Ombudsman shall have the same qualifications as a witness under Section 1.03.

§1.06 REVOCATION

A Directive may be revoked at any time by the declarant, without regard to his or her mental state or competency, by any of the following methods:

(a) By being canceled, defaced, obliterated, burned, torn, or otherwise destroyed by or at the direction of the declarant with the intent to revoke the Directive.

(b) By a written revocation of the declarant expressing his or her intent to revoke the Directive, signed and dated by the declarant. If the declarant is in a health care facility and under the care and management of a physician, the physician shall record in the patient's medical record the time and date when he or she received notification of the written revocation.

(c) By a verbal expression by the declarant of his or her intent to revoke the Directive. The revocation shall become effective only upon communication to the attending physician by the declarant. The attending physician shall confirm with the patient that he or she wishes to revoke, and shall record in the patient's medical record the time, date and place of the revocation.

There shall be no criminal, civil, or administrative liability on the part of any health care provider for following a Directive that has been revoked unless that person has actual knowledge of the revocation.

§1.07 TERM OF DIRECTIVE

A Directive shall be effective unless and until revoked in the manner prescribed in §1.06. This title shall not prevent a declarant from re-executing a Directive at any time in accordance with Section 1.03, including re-execution subsequent to a diagnosis of a terminal condition.   This Directive alone does not permit active voluntary euthanasia. It must be followed by a direct request of the physician as provided for in §1.08.

§1.08 ADMINISTRATION OF AID-IN-DYING

When, and only when, a qualified patient determines that the time for active voluntary euthanasia has arrived and has made an enduring request with a 24 hour waiting period, the patient will communicate that determination directly to the attending physician who will administer euthanasia in accordance with this Act.

§1.09 NO COMPULSION

Nothing herein requires a physician to administer aid-in-dying, or a licensed health care professional, such as a nurse, to participate in administering aid-in-dying under the direction of a physician, if he or she is religiously, morally or ethically opposed. Neither shall privately owned hospitals be required to permit the administration of physician aid-in-dying in their facilities if they are religiously, morally or ethically opposed. Only a physician may carry out this procedure; it may not be delegated to another health professional or person.

§1.10 PROTECTION OF HEALTH CARE PROFESSIONALS

No physician, health care facility or employee of a health care facility who, acting in accordance with the requirements of this title, administers or is present at the administration of active voluntary euthanasia to a qualified patient shall be subject to civil, criminal, or administrative liability therefore. No licensed health care professional, such as a nurse or a pharmacist, acting under the direction of a physician, who participates in the administration of aid-in-dying to a qualified patient in accordance with this title shall be subject to any civil, criminal, or administrative liability. No physician, or licensed health care professional acting under the direction of a physician, who acts in accordance with the provisions of this chapter, shall be guilty of any criminal act or of unprofessional conduct because he or she was present when the aid-in-dying was effected.

§1.11 TRANSFER OF PATIENT

No physician, or health care professional or health care provider acting under the direction of a physician, shall be criminally, civilly, or administratively liable for failing to effectuate the Directive of the qualified patient, unless there is willful failure to agree to transfer the patient to any physician, health care professional, or health care provider upon request of the patient. Refusal to transfer a patient who requests it shall constitute a misdemeanor offense.

§1.12 FEES

Fees, if any, for administering aid-in-dying shall be fair and reasonable.

§1.13 INDEPENDENT PHYSICIANS

The certifying physicians to active voluntary euthanasia shall not be partners or shareholders in the same medical practice. A health maintenance organization shall be exempt from this provision.

§1.14   FAMILY NOTIFICATION

The patient requesting active voluntary euthanasia shall be asked to supply details of next of kin so that they may be notified of this request to die. A patient who declines or cannot supply family details shall not for that reason be denied rights under this Act. If there is objection from the family, the patient's wishes shall prevail.

§1.15 CONSULTATIONS

An attending physician who is requested to give active voluntary euthanasia may request a psychiatric or psychological consultation if that physician has any concern about the patient's competence, with the consent of a qualified patient. A patient should realize that failure to agree to a reasonable request for a consultation may jeopardize the chances of his or her request being carried out.

§1.16 DIRECTIVE COMPLIANCE

Prior to administering active voluntary euthanasia to a qualified patient, the attending physician shall take reasonable steps to determine that the Directive has been signed and witnessed, and all steps are in accord with the desires of the patient, expressed in the Directive and in their personal discussions. Absent knowledge to the contrary, a physician or other health care provider may presume the Directive complies with this title and is valid.

§1.17 MEDICAL STANDARDS

No physician shall be required to take any action contrary to reasonable medical standards in administering aid-in-dying.

§1.18 NOT SUICIDE

Requesting and receiving aid-in-dying by a qualified patient in accordance with this title shall not, for any purpose, including life insurance, constitute a suicide.

§1.19 INSURANCE

(a) No insurer doing business in _____
State shall refuse to insure, cancel, refuse to renew, re-assess the risk of an insured, or raise premiums on the basis of whether or not the insured has considered or completed a Directive. No insurer may require or request the insured to disclose whether he or she has executed a Directive.

(b) The making of a Directive pursuant to Section 1.03 shall not restrict, inhibit, or impair in any manner the sale, procurement, issuance or rates of any policy of life, health, or disability insurance, nor shall it affect in any way the terms of an existing policy of life, health or disability insurance. No policy of life, health, or disability insurance shall be legally impaired or invalidated in any manner by the administration of aid-in-dying to an insured qualified patient, notwithstanding any term of the policy to the contrary.

(c) No physician, health care facility, or other health care provider, and no health care service plan, insurer issuing disability, insurance, other insurer, self-insured employee welfare benefit plan, or non-profit hospital service plan shall require any person to execute or prohibit any person from executing a Directive as a condition for being insured for, or receiving, health care services, nor refuse service because of the execution, the existence, or the revocation of a Directive.

(d) A person who, or a corporation, or other business

which, requires or prohibits the execution of a Directive as a condition for being insured for, or receiving, health care services is guilty of a misdemeanor.

(e) No life insurer doing business in _____ State may refuse to pay sums due upon the death of the insured whose death was assisted in accordance with this Act.

§1.20 INDUCEMENT

No patient may be pressured to make a decision to seek aid-in-dying because that patient is a financial, emotional or other burden to his or her family, other persons, or the state. A person who coerces, pressures or fraudulently induces another to execute a Directive under this chapter is guilty of a misdemeanor, or if death occurs as a result of said coercion, pressure or fraud, is guilty of a homicide punishable according to the laws of this state.

§1.21 TAMPERING

Any person who willfully conceals, cancels, defaces, obliterates, or damages the Directive of another without the declarant's consent shall be guilty of a misdemeanor. Any person who falsifies or forges the Directive of another, or willfully conceals or withholds personal knowledge of a revocation as provided in Section 1.06, with the intent to induce aid-in-dying procedures contrary to the wishes of the declarant, and thereby, because of such act, directly causes aid-in-dying to be administered, shall be subject the prosecution for unlawful homicide punishable according to the laws of this state.

§1.22 OTHER RIGHTS

This Act shall not impair or supersede any right or legal responsibility which any person may have regarding the withholding or withdrawal of life-sustaining procedures in any lawful manner.

§1.23 REPORTING

Hospitals and other health care providers who carry out one of the two Directives of a qualified patient shall keep a record of the number of these cases, and report annually to the State Department of Health Services the patient's age, type of illness, the place and the date the Directive was carried out. In all cases, the identity of the patient shall be strictly confidential and shall not be reported. In the event of a complaint about a specific and named case of aid-in-dying, all pertinent Directives, Advance Directives, medical records, witness statements, and any other evidence must be immediately made available to a review body as appointed by the State Attorney General.

§1.24 RECORDING

The Directive, or a copy of the Directive, shall be made a part of a patient's medical record in each institution involved in the patient's medical care.

§1.25 MERCY KILLING DISAPPROVED

Nothing in this Act shall be construed to condone, authorize, or approve the deliberate ending of a life without the patient's documented and witnessed request.

§1.26 SUICIDE CLINICS

Clinics or centers for the sole purpose of assisting suicide, allowing suicide to take place on the premises, or for the practice of euthanasia shall not be permitted in this state.

§1.27 SEVERABILITY

Any article or section of this Act being held invalid as to any person or circumstance shall not affect the application of any other article or section of this Act which can be given full effect without the invalid article, section, or application.

§1.28 FORM OF DIRECTIVE

In order for a Directive to be valid under this title, the Directive shall be in substantially the following form:

PHYSICIAN-ASSISTED SUICIDE DIRECTIVE

Request to my physician for a prescription for lethal drugs

I hereby request you, my treating physician, _____M.D., to write for me a prescription for lethal drugs which I intend to use to take my life.

This is done in the knowledge we both possess that I am terminally ill and have exhausted all medical procedures acceptable to me.

I acknowledge that you have fully explained to me all available alternatives, including psychological counseling.

I take the legal and moral responsibility for this request to be helped to die, and do hereby absolve you from any legal or administrative culpability.

The time and place of my death will be entirely my personal decision and you need not be involved unless we agree that you will be present.

If I change my mind and do not bring my life to an end I undertake to return either the prescription or the drugs to you for destruction.

Signed _____

Place and Date _____

Witness _____

Place and Date_____

VOLUNTARY DIRECTIVE TO PHYSICIANS
FOR ACTIVE EUTHANASIA

Notice to Patient:

This document will exist until it is revoked by you. This document revokes any prior Directive to administer aid-in-dying but does not revoke a durable power of attorney for health care or living will. You must follow the witnessing procedures described at the end of this form or the document will not be valid. You may wish to give your doctor a signed copy.

INSTRUCTIONS FOR PHYSICIANS

Administration of a Medical Procedure to End My Life in a Painless, Humane, and Dignified Manner

This Directive is made this _____ (day) of _____ (month) _____(year). I, _____, being of sound mind, do voluntarily make known my desire that my life shall be ended with the aid of a physician in a painless, humane, and dignified manner when I have a terminal condition or illness, certified to be terminal by two physicians, and they determine that my death will occur within six months or less. When the terminal diagnosis is made and confirmed, and this Directive is in effect, I may then ask my attending physician for active voluntary euthanasia in the physical presence of two witnesses who are not physicians. I trust and hope that he or she will comply. If he or she refuses to comply, which is his or her right, then I

148

urge that he or she assist in locating a colleague who will comply.

Determining the time and place of my death shall be in my sole discretion. The manner of my death shall be determined jointly be my attending physician and myself. I agree that there shall be present two witnesses who are not physicians when my final request is made for a humane, medically assisted death.

This Directive shall remain valid until revoked by me. I may revoke this Directive at any time.

I recognize that a physician's judgment is not always certain, and that medical science continues to make progress in extending life, but in spite of these facts, I nevertheless wish euthanasia rather than letting my terminal condition take its natural course.

I will endeavor to inform my family of this Directive, and my intention to request the aid of my physician to help me to die when I am in a terminal condition, and take those opinions into consideration. But the final decision remains mine. I acknowledge that it is solely my responsibility to inform my family of my intentions.

I have given full consideration to and understand the full import of this Directive, and I am emotionally and mentally competent to make this Directive. I accept the moral and legal responsibility for receiving euthanasia.

NOTES

This Directive will not be valid unless it is signed by two qualified witnesses who are present when you sign or acknowl-

edge your signature. The witnesses must not be related to you by blood, marriage, or adoption; they must not be entitled to any part of your estate or at the time of execution of the Directive, have no claim against any portion of your estate; and they must not include: your attending physician, an employee of the attending physician; a health care provider; an employee of a health care provider; the operator of the community care facility or an employee of an operator of a community care facility.

If you have attached any additional pages to this form, you must sign and date each of the additional pages at the same time you date and sign this Directive.

Signed: (Name) _____

(City and State of Residence) _____

STATEMENT OF WITNESSES
TO VOLUNTARY DIRECTIVE TO PHYSICIANS

I declare under penalty of perjury under the laws of _____ (State) that the person who signed or acknowledged this document is personally known to me (or proved to me on the basis of satisfactory evidence to be the declarant of this Directive; that he or she signed and acknowledged this Directive in my presence, that he or she appears to be of sound mind and under no duress, fraud, or undue influence; that I am not the attending physician, an employee of the attending physician, a health care provider, an employee of a health care provider, the operator of a community care facility, or an employee of an operator of a community care facility.

I further declare under penalty of perjury under the laws of _____ (State) that I am not related to the declarant by blood, marriage, or adoption, and, to the best of my knowledge, I am not entitled to any part of the estate of the principal upon the death of the principal under a will now existing or by operation of law, and have no claim nor anticipate making a claim against any portion of the estate of the declarant upon his or her death.

Dated: _____

Witness's Signature: _____

Print Name: _____

Residence Address: _____

Dated: _____

Witness's Signature: _____

Print Name: _____

Residence Address: _____

STATEMENT OF PATIENT ADVOCATE
OR OMBUDSMAN

(If you are a patient in a skilled nursing facility, one of the witnesses must be a Patient Advocate or Ombudsman. The following statement is required only if you are a patient in a skilled nursing facility, a health care facility that provides the following basic services: skilled nursing care and supportive care to patients whose primary need is for availability of skilled nursing care on an extended basis. The Patient Advocate or Ombudsman must sign the "Statement of Witnesses" above AND must also sign the following statement.)

I further declare under penalty of perjury under the laws of _____ State that I am a Patient Advocate or Ombudsman as designated by the State Department of Aging and that I am serving as a witness as required by Section _____ of the State Civil Code.

Signed: _____

Date: _____

This Uniform Model Death with Dignity Act is free of copyright.

CALIFORNIA PROPOSITION 161 RESULTS

	YES	%	NO	%
Alameda	235,577	50	235,502	50
Alpine	369	60	244	40
Amador	6,787	47	7,567	53
Butte	37,645	46	43,713	54
Calaveras	5,547	45	6902	35
Colusa	2,266	41	3205	59
Contra Costa	164,671	48	180433	52
Del Norte	4,650	51	4411	49
El Dorado	29,508	49	30660	51
Fresno	76,666	40	113,114	60
Glenn	3,441	40	5202	60
Humboldt	25,788	49	26,691	51
Imperial	9,247	37	15,546	63
Inyo	3,705	48	4064	52
Kern	59,659	37	102204	63
Kings	8,530	37	14693	63
Lake	11,109	49	11342	51
Lassen	4,717	48	5201	52
Los Angeles	1,093,908	45	1,344,144	55
Madera	10,694	37	18579	63
Marin	69,812	60	46,623	40
Mariposa	3,811	48	4095	52
Mendocino	18,481	53	16,404	47
Merced	16,398	37	28,395	63

	YES	%	NO	%
Modoc	2,066	47	2344	53
Mono	2,848	63	1585	37
Monterey	51,202	48	55,311	52
Napa	23,260	46	26,838	54
Nevada	20,875	52	19,604	48
Orange	353,604	42	494,293	58
Placer	35,891	45	43,645	55
Plumas	5,071	50	5059	50
Riverside	160,691	42	226,284	58
Sacramento	179,011	44	224,820	56
San Benito	5,470	45	6625	55
San Bernardino	166,728	40	253,421	60
San Diego	408,186	48	445,087	52
San Francisco	175,691	61	113,114	39
San Joaquin	54,829	40	83,701	60
San Luis Obispo	47,964	50	48,887	50
San Mateo	120,341	50	120,407	50
Santa Barbara	67,958	47	76,107	53
Santa Clara	261,515	49	275,431	51
Santa Cruz	57,411	56	44,815	44
Shasta	26,015	40	38,309	60
Sierra	912	50	911	50
Siskiyou	9,792	49	10,395	51
Solano	53,754	44	67,881	56
Sonoma	92,818	53	83,730	47
Stanislaus	39,899	37	68,121	63
Sutter	9,842	40	14,766	60
Tehama	8,838	43	11,887	57
Trinity	3,343	52	3,082	48
Tulare	28,911	35	54,151	65

Tuolomne	9,507	43	12,840	57
Ventura	140,169	56	107,988	44
Yolo	27,899	49	29,128	51
Yuba	7,013	42	9,658	58
Totals	**4,562,010**	**46**	**5,348,947**	**54**

59 precincts total in California
5 were tied at 50-50
11 were won outright

Eleven doctors accused in the USA

Eleven doctors have been charged with killing a terminally ill patient or family member. None, however, has been sent to prison. The cases are:

1935

A general practitioner in Montevista, Colorado, **Harold Blazer**, was accused of the murder of his thirty year-old daughter, Hazel, a victim of cerebral spinal meningitis. Evidence was given that she had the mind of a baby and her limbs were the size of a five year-old child. Dr. Blazer, together with his wife and another daughter, had taken care of Hazel for thirty years. One day he placed a handkerchief soaked in chloroform over her face and kept it in place until she died. At his trial, the doctor was acquitted.

1950

New Hampshire doctor **Hermann N. Sanders** was charged with the first degree murder of a terminally ill patient, Abbie Borroto. At the request of Borroto's husband, Sanders injected Borroto with 44 cc's of air and she died within ten minutes. When he logged the fatal injection into the hospital record, Sanders was reported to authorities. At the close of a three week trial, the jury deliberated an hour and ten minutes before returning a verdict of innocent.

1972

Long Island doctor **Vincent Montemarano**, chief surgical resident at the Nassau County Medical Center, was indicted on a charge of willful murder in the death of fifty-nine year-old Eugene Bauer. Bauer, suffering with cancer of the throat, had been given two days to live. Bauer died within five minutes of Montemarano's injection of potassium chloride. The defense argued that the state did not prove Bauer was alive prior to the injection. The jury deliberated fifty-five minutes before returning an innocent verdict.

1981

California doctors **Robert Nedjl** and **Neil Barber** were charged with murder for discontinuing mechanical ventilation and intravenous fluids to Clarence Herbert, aged 55. The patient had a heart attack after surgery to correct an intestinal obstruction. Herbert stayed in a coma for three days before his condition was declared hopeless. Following the wishes of Herbert's wife and eight children, he was taken off life-support systems but continued to breathe. Five days later the intravenous fluid was discontinued. Herbert died six days later. In October, 1983, a court of appeals dismissed the charges.

1985

Dr. John Kraai, an old-time physician from a small New York town, was charged with second degree murder in the death of his patient and friend, Frederick Wagner, 81. Wagner suffered from Alzheimer's disease for five years and had gangrene of the foot. On the morning of Wagner's death, Kraai injected three large doses of insulin into Wagner's chest.

As Wagner's condition worsened, a nurse called the State Department of Patient Abuse. Kraai was charged with murder. Three weeks after his arrest, Kraai killed himself with a lethal injection.

1986

New Jersey doctor **Joseph Hassman** was charged with murder in connection with the death of his mother-in-law, Esther Davis, 80, who suffered from Alzheimer's disease. At the family's request, Hassmann injected Davis with a lethal dose of Demerol. Hassman cried several times in court during the trial. He was found guilty and sentenced to two years probation, fined $10,000 and ordered to perform four hundred hours of community service.

1987

Fort Myers doctor **Peter Rosier** was acquitted of first degree murder in the death of his wife, Patricia. Pat tried to end her life with an overdose of Seconal, but when the powerful sedative did not take hold, Rosier began injecting her with morphine. The morphine was not lethal. Rosier did not then know it, but Pat's stepfather, Vincent Delman smothered her.

1989

Dr Donald Caraccio, 33, of Troy, Michigan, was charged in Detroit with the murder of a 74-year-old woman hospital patient who was terminally ill and comatose. Dr.

Caraccio gave the patient a lethal injection of potassium chloride in the presence of other medical staff. In court, the doctor said he did it to terminate her pain and suffering. Evidence was given that he was overworked and stressed by the recent lengthy and painful death of his father. Accepting Dr. Caraccio's guilty plea, the judge imposed five years probation with community service.

1990

Dr. Richard Schaeffer, 69, was arrested under suspicion of having caused the death by injection at the home of a patient, Melvin Seifert, 75, of Redondo Beach, California, who was suffering from the effects of a stroke and other ailments. The dead man's wife, Mary, 75, was also arrested. Both were released pending further investigation, and a year later it was announced that there would be no charges.

1990

Dr. Jack Kevorkian was charged in December with the first degree murder of Hemlock Society member Janet Adkins who died on June 4. Suffering from Alzheimer's disease, Mrs. Adkins flew from her home in Portland, Oregon, to Michigan, where Dr. Kevorkian connected her to his so-called "suicide machine." She chose the time to press a button which resulted in lethal drugs entering her body. Ten days after being charged, a court dismissed the murder charge.

1992

Dr. Kevorkian was charged with two counts of murder and delivery of a controlled substance for the October 23, 1991 deaths of Marjorie Wantz, 58, and Sherry Miller, 43. Both women were chronically ill-- Miller suffered from multiple sclerosis and Wantz had chronic pelvic pain. Sherry Miller used the "suicide machine" to commit suicide. Marjorie Wantz inhaled carbon monoxide through a mask. Oakland County (Michigan) Circuit Judge David Breck dismissed the murder charges when the prosecution was unable to prove that Kevorkian tripped the devices that killed the women.

Bibliography

Suggested readings on legal aspects of physician-assisted suicide

Journals

Battin, Margaret. "Assisted Suicide: Can we learn from Germany?" _Hastings Center Report._ v22, n2. p44-51.

Brandt, Craig and Patricia Cone, et al. "Model aid-in-dying act" _Iowa Law Review._ v75, n1. p125-215.

de Wachter, Maurice A.M. "Euthanasia in the Netherlands." _Hastings Center Report._ v22, n2. p23-30.

Drey, Paul and James Giszczak. "May I author my final chapter? Assisted suicide and guidelines to prevent abuse." _Journal of Legislation._ Summer 1992. v18. p331-345.

Nerland, Lynn Tracy. "A cry for help: A comparison of voluntary, active euthanasia law." _Hastings International and Comparative Law Review._ v13. Fall 1989. p115-139.

Pletcher, Robert A. "Assisted suicide for the terminally ill: the inadequacy of current legal models to rationally analyze voluntary active euthanasia." _Criminal Justice Journal._ v13. Spring 1992. p303-317.

Reno, Juliana. "A little help from my friends: the legal status of assisted suicide." *Creighton Law Review*. v25. June 1992. p1151-1183.

Smith, George P. II. "All's well that ends well: toward a policy of assisted rational suicide or merely enlightened self-determination?" (Symposium of Law and Medicine) *UC Davis Law Review*. v22. Winter 89. p275-419.

Books

Connelly, Robert J. PhD. *Last Rights: Death and dying in Texas law and experience.* Corona Publishing Co. 1992.

Humphry, Derek and Ann Wickett. *The Right to Die: Understanding euthanasia.* Harper and Row. New York. 1986.

Meisel, Alan. *The Right to Die.* Wiley Law Publications. New York. 1992.

Risley, Robert L. J.D. *Death with Dignity: A new law permitting physician aid-in-dying.* National Hemlock Society. Eugene, Oregon. 1989.

Rosenblatt, Stanley M. *Murder of Mercy: Euthanasia on Trial.* Prometheus Books. Buffalo, New York. 1992.

Organizations Directly Concerned With Changing The Law on Physician aid-in-dying

AMERICANS FOR DEATH WITH DIGNITY
(Formerly Americans/Californians Against Human Suffering)
Founded 1986 by Robert Risley

Political campaigners. Nonprofit but not tax deductible. Sole aim is to change the law, first in California and then throughout America, to permit physician aid-in-dying.

> P O Box 11001
> Glendale CA 91226

CITIZENS FOR PATIENT SELF-DETERMINATION
(Formerly Washington Citizens for Death With Dignity)
Founded 1990

Political campaigners. Nonprofit but not tax deductible. Fights for all rights of terminally ill persons living in Washington State, particularly physician aid-in-dying.

> P O Box 84463
> Seattle   WA 98124

HEMLOCK SOCIETY (OREGON) INC.
Founded 1987 by Derek Humphry

Political campaigners. Nonprofit but not tax deductible. Seeks lawful physician aid-in-dying in the state of Oregon by voters' initiative.

PO Box 25075
Portland   OR 97225-0075

PATIENTS' RIGHTS ORGANIZATION OF FLORIDA, INC.

Founded 1993
Political campaigners. Nonprofit but not tax deductible.
A coalition of the 15 Hemlock chapters in Florida, P R O F coordinates political efforts to reach legislators and voters, gives testimony at legislative hearings, and does lobbying.

P O Box 31142
Sarasota FL 34232-0142

166

Books on the right to choose
to die by Derek Humphry

FINAL EXIT: The practicalities of self-deliverance and assisted suicide for the dying.
Every person who cares about control and choice in dying should have this classic on their bookshelf. It outlines each step a dying person may need to take to commit suicide if the suffering is unbearable. Clear advice about the law on assisted suicide is given, plus precise drug details. *Final Exit* was 18 weeks on the *New York Times* bestseller list, has sold more than 600,000 copies in North America, and been translated into eleven major languages. This is the 1992 updated edition.

Dell Paperbacks $10.00
ISBN 0-440-50488-0

JEAN'S WAY
The story of Jean Humphry's battle against cancer and how her husband helped her end her life has become a cult classic, constantly published worldwide since 1978. The attention which this book received launched the Hemlock Society. The *San Francisco Examiner* called it "A tender and rare love story which will touch every reader."

Dell Paperbacks $4.99
ISBN 0-440-21295-2

DYING WITH DIGNITY: Understanding euthanasia.
The cream of Derek Humphry's essays on euthanasia are collected in this 1992 book. Written in plain, non-jargon language, they explain the background to the *cause celebre* mercy killing cases in America, and the uphill fight to change the law in America to permit lawful physician aid-in-dying for the terminally ill.

Carol Publishing   Hardcover $16.95
ISBN 1-55972-105-7

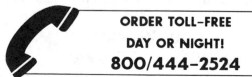

ORDER TOLL-FREE
DAY OR NIGHT!
800/444-2524

Lawful Exit

$9.95
A paperback original
(not published in hardcover)
ISBN 0-9637280-0-8

Published by:

The Norris Lane Press
24829 Norris Lane
Junction City OR 97448-9559

Telephone and fax: 503/998-1873

Distributed to the book and library trade by:

BookWorld Services, Inc.
1993 Whitfield Loop
Sarasota FL 34243

Telephone: 800/444-2524 anytime
Fax: 813/753-9396

<u>**Personal credit card telephone orders:**</u>
(VISA, MasterCard, Discover and American Express)

BookWorld
1-800-444-2524